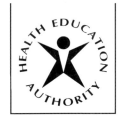

Effectiveness of physical activity promotion schemes in primary care: a review

Chris Riddoch
Anna Puig-Ribera
and Ashley Cooper
Exercise and Health Research Unit
University of Bristol

HEA Project Team

Alana Diamond   Research Project Manager

In the same series:

Health promotion in older people for the prevention of coronary heart disease and stroke

Health promotion in childhood and young adolescence for the prevention of unintentional injuries

Effectiveness of video for health education: a review

Effectiveness of mental health promotion interventions: a review

Health promotion with young people for the prevention of substance misuse

Health promotion interventions to promote healthy eating in the general population

Effectiveness of oral health promotion

Effectiveness of interventions to promote healthy eating in pre-school children aged 1–5 years: a review

Effectiveness of interventions to promote healthy eating in elderly people living in the community: a review

Effectiveness of interventions to promote healthier living in people from minority ethnic groups: a review

Effectiveness of interventions to promote healthy eating in pregnant women and women of childbearing age: a review

ISBN 0 7521 1283 X

Health Education Authority
Trevelyan House
30 Great Peter Street
London SW1P 2HW

Designed by Edwin Belchamber
Typeset by Wayzgoose
Cover design by Maria Grasso
Printed in Great Britain

Contents

Acknowledgements

The authors are very grateful for the considerable assistance they have received from the following people, without whose help the report would not have been possible:

- the managers of 'exercise on prescription' schemes for their generous investment of time in the completion of questionnaires, provision of supporting documentation, and great enthusiasm for the concept of this review
- health promotion specialists for their assistance in identification of schemes and co-ordination of data collection
- participants in the three case studies for their contribution of time and other valuable resources which ensured the success of this element of the project
- academic colleagues in the UK and abroad who work in this field of study for the generous provision of papers, data and general advice
- Mrs Pat Turton, Department of Social Medicine, University of Bristol, and Mrs Dawn Vernon, Wiltshire Health Promotion Service, for proofreading an initial draft of this report, and offering insightful comments on the presentation of the report.

Structure of the report

The report begins with commentaries by Nick Cavill from the HEA and Dr Adrian Taylor, Senior Lecturer in Sport and Exercise Psychology at the University of Brighton.

The report is then divided into three main sections: an executive summary, the main report and appendices.

The *executive summary* contains the methodology, the main findings and recommendations for the design and evaluation of schemes.

The *main report* provides a background to the promotion of physical activity in primary care. Details of the methodology and scope of the review are given in Chapter 3. The results of the systematic review are presented in Chapter 4. Case studies conducted to gain a better insight into the impact of schemes are introduced in Chapter 5, along with their methodology. Chapters 6–8 provide the results of the case studies. The results of both the systematic review and the case studies are discussed in Chapter 9, and conclusions presented in Chapter 10. Recommendations for both the design and evaluation of schemes are in Chapter 11. Chapter 12 comments on the implications for the proposed healthy living centres.

The *appendices* provide details of the systematic review methodology and the response categories for the case studies.

Reports cited in this review are identified by the surname of the author(s) and year of publication.

Commentary

Nick Cavill, Programme Manager: physical activity programme, HEA

The principle of 'exercise on prescription' appears to be a simple and attractive one. Instead of simply recommending exercise to patients, primary health care professionals are able to 'prescribe' a programme of exercise, typically delivered through an arrangement with a local leisure centre or other exercise facility. The principle is that the exercise programme will be safe and effective, and that the schemes will increase compliance.

This idea has caught on in recent years, with a mushrooming of schemes in existence. But do they work? Are these schemes effective in promoting increased participation in physical activity, and does this lead to measurable benefits to health?

The HEA commissioned this review to provide an overview of the published scientific evidence of the effectiveness of exercise on prescription schemes. This is important in the current climate where evidence is needed to support funding decisions. In addition to examining the peer-reviewed literature, case studies were conducted on schemes that were perceived to be successful. Hence, the wider impact and determinants of these schemes has also been considered.

This review is not only useful for those who are planning or implementing schemes, but it also raises important research and evaluation issues that should be addressed.

Commentary

Dr Adrian H Taylor, Senior Lecturer in Sport and Exercise Psychology, Chelsea School, University of Brighton

There has been a rapid growth in the promotion of physical activity in the past eight years in the UK, although there is a very mixed interest in 'exercise on prescription' schemes among those working in primary care. There may be a number of reasons for this, such as:

- Practitioners are unable to identify sedentary populations, due to the complexity of measuring physical activity.

- Practitioners do not know enough about the type of physical activity and the recommended dose necessary for health benefits.

- Practitioners have only limited training and skills in behaviour change strategies or counselling. They may also fall into the trap of the self-fulfilling prophecy: that is, previous attempts to change behaviour have resulted in failure, so why attempt to promote change?

- Physical activity tends not to be on patients' agenda when they present to primary care services. Patients may be keener to receive conventional therapeutic interventions to relieve symptoms of ill health.

- Consultation times, averaging just seven minutes per patient, provide little opportunity for GPs to assess a patient's physical activity levels, let alone advise or counsel on physical activity.

This review broadens the debate about how best to promote physical activity through primary-care based initiatives, beyond the traditional role of the general practitioner. It encompasses a review of both the effectiveness of interventions delivered by trained exercise specialists (e.g. counselling), and schemes involving referral to exercise practitioners in leisure facilities.

The primary goal of the review is to inform commissioners, policy analysts, purchasers, providers and lottery fund holders (for healthy living centres), on the effective use of resources in promoting physical activity in primary care.

The review also addresses the professional training and research implications of future promotional activity.

Evidence for the effectiveness of physical activity interventions is based on: a systematic review of UK-based interventions; a systematic review of primary-care based interventions throughout the world; and three case studies of exercise prescription schemes in the UK. This review illuminates the scope of research within the field in a number of ways.

- Very few studies of adequate quality are available to form the basis for a systematic review.

- Most of the studies have been conducted overseas, particularly in North America, and their applicability to the UK context may be very limited (see Hillsdon and Thorogood, 1996; Webborn, 1996).

- A wide range of outcome measures of physical activity and, indeed, fitness, has been used, resulting in contradictory findings in some cases. This makes an effectiveness review difficult to conduct (see Taylor, 1996).

- The economic costs of primary care interventions have rarely been considered (see Stevens et al., 1998), even though the promotion of physical activity has been positively argued for (Morris, 1994; Nichol, 1994). This makes comparison across interventions virtually impossible, since better resources no doubt increase the likelihood of behaviour change.

- Much of the research undertaken in the UK on GP exercise referral programmes has been conducted in-house, by leisure providers with limited resources for robust research. The exercise-referral case studies in the present review paint a rather positive view of effectiveness. A focus on short-term outcomes and patients who stay in a programme will inevitably provide the most positive findings compared with an intent-to-treat analysis.

- Those most at risk or of poorest health status are least likely to enter and adhere to an exercise programme, or indeed a research study. However, some evidence suggests that obese patients are more likely to adhere to a leisure-centre based exercise programme (see Taylor et al., 1998).

Nevertheless, the authors of the review make constructive use of the various research sources available. The document provides a valuable summary of the issues in effectiveness reviews, and opens perhaps as many doors as it closes. While it is not desirable to set a blueprint for healthy living centres, the review provides a framework for cost-effective interventions.

- Primary-care based exercise referral programmes, often involving referral by a GP to a leisure facility, are not necessarily effective in increasing long-term physical activity.

- Effectiveness is likely to be greater in the following circumstances:
  - staff are trained in behaviour change strategies and are sympathetic to the needs of sedentary individuals who may have additional medical needs
  - there is an appropriate exercise practitioner-to-patient ratio, to enable quality supervision and support
  - liaison between health and leisure service personnel is established and maintained
  - a community-based network is established to offer support and interaction during and beyond the referral programme, also incorporating sustainable active living.

- A dose of 30 minutes of accumulated moderate activity, at least five days a week, is justified from a coronary heart disease risk reduction perspective. There are other dose–response relationships between physical activity and different health outcomes (e.g. psychological and osteoporosis risk) which also deserve recognition within a tailored exercise programme.

- Where exercise prescription schemes have been allowed to operate over a period of time (despite recent instability in health and leisure service provision) many lessons have been learnt about improving effectiveness (see Taylor, 1998). A blend of academic and applied expertise should be used to design, implement and evaluate primary care interventions.

In conclusion, this review is welcome for a number of reasons: first, it re-emphasises the importance of physical activity promotion. Second, the review highlights the urgent need for specialist professionals able to provide appropriate exercise programmes, leadership and evaluation expertise. Third, the need for further research in the UK context is clearly identified. Finally, the review broadens the debate about appropriate forms of evaluation (i.e. other than randomised controlled trials) for exercise and health promotion interventions.

Background

Prescription of physical activity is becoming increasingly common within primary care. Within a climate of evidence-based medicine, there is a need to assess the effectiveness of such schemes. Although many schemes exist, few are evaluated in a rigorous manner, although some pilot studies and some larger funded studies are now coming to fruition and data relating to effectiveness are emerging.

Aim

The main aim of this review was to collect and evaluate the evidence relating to primary-care based physical activity promotion schemes within the United Kingdom. More specifically, we have tried to:

- estimate the effectiveness of schemes in promoting increased levels of physical activity and associated factors
- estimate the wider impact of schemes, as perceived by a variety of participants
- compare UK practice with practice elsewhere, specifically the United States
- discuss the implications of the results for practice and policy in this area.

Research questions

Two initial research questions were formulated.

1. What is the effectiveness of primary-care based physical activity promotion programmes with respect to increasing physical activity levels?
2. What is the effectiveness of primary-care based physical activity promotion programmes with respect to modifying mediators of physical activity, and attitudes/intentions towards physical activity?

Three case studies were conducted with a focus on the wider impact of schemes.

Methods

The study comprised: (a) a systematic review of empirical data relating to the effectiveness of schemes, and (b) three case studies of existing schemes.

Systematic review

A systematic search of relevant electronic databases was conducted from their year of inception to 1998. Known books, book chapters, and reviews were searched visually. Reference lists of retrieved articles were also searched visually. Hand searching of key journals was undertaken to identify studies not yet indexed. Known authors in the field were contacted by letter asking for information, further analyses, papers 'in press' and for further information which would be useful for the review. Follow-up letters and telephone calls were made to non-responders as appropriate. Questionnaires requesting data on internal evaluations were sent to scheme managers, to be supported by additional documentation where appropriate.

Inclusion criteria were established as:

- studies of adults (> 16 years)
- aim of study to improve physical activity levels, mediators of physical activity, or attitudes/intentions towards physical activity
- initiated within a primary care setting
- physical activity or related measure was an identifiable outcome measure or focus
- UK-based.

Each identified study was assessed for quality independently, on a five-point scale.

Case studies

Three case studies were conducted of schemes of varied geographical location, activity 'prescriptions' and messages, and settings for activity. Data collection lasted an average of 4 days and included semi-structured interviews, document searches, informal discussions, shadowing of key personnel, and observational techniques.

The focus of the case studies was on the perceptions of effectiveness and the overall level of impact, beyond the specific effects on referred patients. Included in this were potential effects on scheme administrators, doctors, nurses, leisure centre staff and families of patients. Where possible, data were collected from local authority personnel, scheme organisers, physicians, and exercise referral specialists. For confidentiality and ethical reasons no data were collected from patients.

Results

Systematic review

- Two hundred and fifty-four papers relating to some aspect of physical activity promotion in primary care were identified. Twenty-five papers were identified as being empirical in nature, and of these twelve satisfied the five inclusion criteria for the review.

- No large-scale randomised controlled trials using physical activity as the main outcome measure have been conducted in the UK, most studies being relatively small scale. The few large-scale studies attempt to modify classical risk factors, using physical activity as one of a number of intermediary factors.

- The majority of studies report some form of improvement in either physical activity or related measures. However, the size of the effect is generally small, and there is limited consistency across studies. Non-UK studies were reviewed for comparative purposes, and similar effects were observed.

- Given the diversity of design and the limited power of most studies, it is encouraging to observe positive, albeit limited, effects. Isolation of such effects is an achievement given the complexity and difficulty of measuring physical activity behaviour. Most studies adopt an experimental approach, using a small number of outcomes, including physical activity. Such an approach provides valuable information, but gives no information on the wider impact of schemes.

Grey literature

- Forty-five sets of documentation were received from scheme managers.

- Forty-one schemes (93%) are undertaking some form of evaluation. Research methodology, however, is consistently flawed. Many schemes report that no data are yet available. Where data are available, a diverse range of effects is reported, nearly all of which are positive. In some cases the level of effect is very large. These data suggest a much greater level of effect compared to the published studies, but study design is usually very weak and only a limited degree of emphasis can be afforded to these data.

- Although a few schemes report the use of a psychological model of behaviour change, this is rather rare, and in no case are details of the model or strategy available.

Case studies

- Data from case studies suggest a higher level, and more diverse, impact. Schemes are perceived to have an impact not only upon the patients, but also on primary care staff, leisure centre staff, communities, and friends and colleagues of all involved. Effects on patients are perceived to be principally in the social and psychological domains.

- All three schemes are perceived as very successful, despite being diverse in location, setting and organisation. Common factors which appear to consistently contribute to the success of these schemes are: staff enthusiasm, working within alliances and maintaining good communications between the organisations, designing individual exercise programmes tailored to each patient's needs and having individual supervision, and having a low-cost policy, especially in areas of low income.

- Being a member of a scheme appears important, for social and psychological reasons. Even very small achievements in these respects are perceived as meaningful. Patients find support, a social life, and self-confidence. Patients experience an improved quality of life. Patients suffering from anxiety or depression are seen to benefit particularly. Individualised prescriptions and supervision are seen as important factors, particularly for patients who are initially fearful of exercise.

- The fixed length of programmes means that effects are normally short term, unless a continuing strategy is available for patients at the end of the programme.

Main conclusions

- Published studies demonstrate small but possibly meaningful improvements in physical activity patterns and other activity-related measures. In contrast, data from the case studies suggest considerable impact in a range of parameters and on a variety of people. The discrepancy between the results of the two approaches raises important questions as to future research strategies and how we should interpret the evidence.

- Systematic gathering of quality data across the many existing schemes, using valid measures, would provide substantial evidence relating to effectiveness. In particular, the potential high volume of data would ensure that sufficient statistical power is obtained to detect small effects. Careful selection of outcomes and methodology would ensure that data gathering is cost-effective and not too onerous for staff. Such evaluations should be accompanied by relevant training in evaluation procedures.

- As far as we can detect, no existing UK programmes are based on an accepted model of behaviour change.

- The role of the leisure centre as a setting for activity promotion may be problematical, and needs a conceptual review. It may be that the projected 'healthy living centres' are more appropriate settings.

- Expectations of programme success should be realistic. Major changes in large numbers of participants are unlikely to happen. However, small but positive effects are meaningful when large numbers of people experience them.

Implications

Physical activity is relatively new on the heath promotion agenda, and significant cultural shifts in society are required before one can expect large-scale changes in behaviour. Supporting environmental initiatives may also be required. The small but positive effects revealed in this review must be viewed within this context, and it may be unrealistic to expect large-scale changes in behaviour at such an early stage in the promotion of physical activity. For example, smoking cessation interventions have been in existence for over 20 years, and yet only recently have there been substantial shifts in behaviour.

Implications for the design and implementation of schemes

- The large majority of current schemes are facility based, and yet it is not clear if the literature supports this strategy, especially in terms of uptake and adherence to programmes. Home and community-based settings might in future be considered as more appropriate for many referred patients, as they carry fewer sport/fitness-orientated connotations. The proposed healthy living centres, which will be community-based, may have an important role to play in the future of exercise on prescription schemes.

- It may be prudent for schemes to adopt and promote the physical activity recommendation for general health, i.e. half an hour of moderate intensity physical activity a day. This message is more flexible than the traditional recommendation for cardiovascular and muscular fitness. The moderate message may be more appropriate for use in non-facility settings and with a wider range of population groups.

- It is of crucial importance that training for, and the organisation of schemes (including patient selection, programme design, materials and programme delivery) are theoretically based and utilise what we know to be successful. There are clear indications in the literature that certain strategies are more successful than others, and it is essential that this forms the basis upon which all schemes are built.

○ Appropriate training of both primary care and referral staff in relevant theory-led techniques (such as counselling and motivational interviewing) is needed, to maximise patient motivation. Appropriate training for exercise referral specialists is vital to the success and safety of schemes. The typical sports science qualification concentrates largely on physically training the young and healthy individual, whereas in reality the individuals referred on to schemes can be older, less healthy, and lacking in motivation for physical activity.

Implications for the evaluation of schemes

○ Virtually all the published literature is experimental. While such methodologies are important, in that they isolate the primary outcome measure – physical activity participation – they tend to ignore the wider social impact of schemes. A pluralistic approach to evaluation, with outcome measures that include psycho-social variables, may provide a more accurate estimation of the true impact of schemes.

○ Physical activity is notoriously difficult to measure, and many internal evaluations as well as published trials have used questionnaires of dubious validity and reliability. Many existing questionnaires are biased towards the estimation of sport and exercise, as opposed to moderate activities such as housework and gardening, which may contribute *subtly* but significantly to increased participation. Future studies should use valid and reliable questionnaires, and objective validation using motion sensors should also be considered.

○ Physical activity level is an important outcome measure for any effectiveness study. However, many referred patients are not expected to change activity level, at least in the short term. It may be that the assessment of mediators of physical activity (e.g. self-efficacy, Stage of Change) are an appropriate additional outcome measure for many patients who may be 'on the way' to behaviour change.

○ The transient health effects of activity mean that the ultimate goal of schemes should be long-term participation in an active lifestyle. However, many evaluations only carry a pre-post analysis – typically over a time period of just a few months. Some schemes have used a 26-week follow-up, but longer periods are rare. Longer-term follow-up is essential in order to assess meaningful health gain.

1. Introduction

The aim of this review is to assess the effectiveness of UK primary-care based physical activity promotion schemes. Such schemes are proliferating, with a previous review identifying 121 schemes (Biddle, Fox and Edmunds, 1994). In a 1996 directory of GP-referral schemes (Chapman, 1996) the author states that there are (in 1996) at least 200 schemes, and probably many more. For this reason, and also with the increasing emphasis being placed on the way we live our lives as a means of improving public health (Department of Health, 1992 and 1998), the review is timely.

There is no doubt that sedentary lifestyles are a major health-related problem in the UK (Health Education Authority and Sports Council, 1992), a situation which also exists in other industrialised nations, and initiatives to increase physical activity levels will come under increased scrutiny both in terms of organisation and effectiveness.

Previous reviews of the effectiveness of primary-care based physical activity promotion schemes have been conducted.* Some of these (Ashenden, Silagy and Weler, 1997; Hillsdon and Thorogood, 1996; Hillsdon et al., 1995) have focused on the results of randomised controlled trials, whereas others (Dishman and Buckworth, 1996) have adopted a more inclusive approach. There are clear indications in this literature that physical activity promotion programmes, in a variety of forms, can be successful. However, within these reviews UK studies of effectiveness are scarce, and they contain no UK studies which have been conducted within a primary care setting.

In a climate of evidence-based medicine it is unfortunate that such a popular public health initiative does not currently have a firm foundation of evidence from which effectiveness can be judged. However, we are aware that a few of the larger schemes are being evaluated in a more rigorous manner. Further, we are aware that some schemes incorporate systematic data gathering and evaluation procedures which can potentially be used to monitor progress. However, such evaluations often address the process aspects, rather than the patient-specific outcomes of the scheme.

*See Ashenden, Silagy and Weler, 1997; Biddle, Fox and Edmunds, 1994; Dishman and Buckworth, 1996; Dunn, 1996; Eaton and Menard, 1998; Hillsdon and Thorogood, 1996; Hillsdon et al., 1995; Marcus et al., 1995.

This is not surprising, as rigorous assessment of the effects on participants is a difficult task, requiring detailed knowledge of research design and measurement issues, not least when the outcome measure of most interest, physical activity, is a complex behaviour which is difficult to measure. This level of evaluation requires specialist input, and without collaboration with a recognised research organisation, it is normally beyond the scope of most scheme managers. Rigorous evaluation therefore relies heavily on a partnership with a research organisation and on external research funding.

It is now clear, however, that in the UK evidence relating to the effectiveness of schemes is accumulating, and there currently exists a coherent body of evidence which can be used to gain a measure of effectiveness. In a climate of increasingly scarce resources there is a need for evidence-based health promotion, and we feel that this body of evidence is now worthy of evaluation.

Physical activity and health

Physical activity is now accepted as a major contributor to good health (Department of Health and Human Services, 1996), and an increasingly important focus for health promotion. Evidence from epidemiological studies clearly indicates that morbidity and mortality from a range of chronic diseases are lower in physically active groups compared to sedentary groups (Powell *et al.*, 1987). This relationship is particularly noticeable for coronary heart disease (CHD), which is twice as common in inactive groups compared to active groups (Powell *et al.*, 1987). The level of increased risk seen in sedentary populations is comparable to levels of risk resulting from hypertension, cigarette smoking and high blood cholesterol concentrations (Berlin and Colditz, 1990; Powell *et al.*, 1987). Further, modern, inactive lifestyles are thought to be at least as important as diet in the aetiology of obesity and possibly represent the dominant factor (Prentice and Jebb, 1995). Physical inactivity has therefore been acknowledged by the American Heart Association as a major risk factor for CHD (Fletcher *et al.*, 1992). Regular physical activity can also help prevent non-insulin dependent diabetes mellitus, hypertension, osteoporosis, mental health problems and obesity. Some forms of cancer and stroke are also less prevalent in active groups.

There is no doubt that today's high level of mechanisation in transport, and both home and occupational work fosters sedentary living patterns, and in the UK a high prevalence of sedentary behaviour has been identified, with 70–90% of men and women being insufficiently active to achieve health benefits (Health Education Authority and Sports Council, 1992). Accordingly, the promotion of physical activity is becoming a public health issue of increasing importance.

The health benefits of physical activity are transient. In other words, physical activity only confers health benefits during the stages of life when an active lifestyle is adopted. For example, Paffenbarger *et al.* (1993) have demonstrated that adopting an active lifestyle later in life is related independently to prolonged life. Similarly, Blair *et al.* (1995) have reported that adults who achieved improved aerobic fitness over a five-year period demonstrated reduced risk of CHD. The 'protective' effect of activity must be mediated by physiological changes, although the precise mechanisms have yet to be detected. It is logical to presume that these changes are reversible should the active lifestyle cease. The implications of this are clear – the health benefits of physical activity are available throughout adult life, and will be lost should sedentary living be resumed.

Exercise prescription for health

Of major significance for those who prescribe physical activity for health purposes is the significant 'paradigm shift' concerning what constitutes a healthy level of activity (Blair, 1995). In particular, there is increasing recognition that vigorous, fitness training activity, while probably healthy in most cases, is not *required* in order to achieve a health benefit. It is now recognised that more moderate activities, equating to brisk walking, confer substantial health benefit. Importantly, such activities are more attractive and sustainable for more people. Indeed there is evidence to suggest that 10-minute exercise sessions are equally efficacious in improving both fitness and health parameters compared to longer sessions (DeBusk *et al.*, 1990; Murphy and Hardman, 1998).

It should be considered that the physiological changes which promote improved health probably involve haemostatic and biochemical changes, for example improved lipid profile, clotting factors, improved glucose tolerance, reduced blood pressure. The key question which underpins exercise prescription is what type and level of activity is most effective in modifying these various factors. Whereas it is not possible to answer this question from experimental data, two key factors emerge from the epidemiological evidence. Firstly, the key dimension of physical activity which confers health benefits is the *volume* of activity, irrespective of the duration of activity bouts, the number of activity bouts per week, and possibly the intensity of the activity (Blair, 1995). Secondly, the most dramatic reduction in risk is between the most sedentary individuals and those in the next highest activity category. Again this carries considerable implications for activity promotion schemes in terms of the activity 'messages' which are given. More moderate activity carries the majority of health benefits and is behaviourally more sustainable.

It is well documented that different 'doses' of activity can have differing responses (Haskell, 1994). This has important ramifications in that just as patients are likely to differ in age, disease status and goals, so the activity 'prescription' must vary. This is important in terms of both safety and effectiveness. It is also related closely to the knowledge, expertise and qualifications of the physical activity referral specialist, who needs to know the dangers and benefits of physical activity, in all its forms, in a wide variety of clinical conditions. In this respect, the related issues of training of referral specialists and liability are bound to assume increasing importance.

Determinants of physical activity

Psychological factors are related in important ways to both uptake of activity and long-term adherence to the 'programme' or an active lifestyle, and act in concert with personal characteristics and environmental factors (Marcus, 1995). Each of these should be considered when developing an activity promotion programme. For example, consideration of personal characteristics (for example age, sex, ethnicity, body size) may be important for the effective targeting of participants; psychological variables (for example self-efficacy, perceived health status, motivation) may influence the style of delivery; and environmental factors (for example social support, costs, location) might influence the setting of the activity and the specific characteristics of the programme. King *et al.* (1995) have further argued that policy, legislative, regulatory, and environmental interventions are all important facets of any physical activity campaign to prevent cardiovascular disease (CVD) and other chronic diseases.

A particular problem is that many individuals have very good intentions to become more active, and many do try to become more active. However, the general pattern is that the majority find insuperable barriers and eventually relapse into their previous sedentary lifestyle. Given that the health benefits of activity are transient, no health gain is achieved. It is common to see low levels of uptake of activity programmes, and up to 50% drop-out from programmes within 6–12 months (King *et al.*, 1992).

In addition to the above factors, it has further been suggested that the support of the family physician could be a powerful additional element in the individual's support network for adopting and maintaining an active lifestyle (Anderson *et al.*, 1997).

Guidelines for health-related physical activity

In the light of the above, health-related activity guidelines have been published for American adults (Pate *et al.*, 1995), and for UK adults (Department of Health, 1996). Each broadly emphasises 30 minutes of moderate intensity (equivalent to brisk walking) activity on at least 5 days of the week. This is a major shift from previous guidelines which emphasised cardiovascular fitness training, and demanded three sessions of vigorous activity per week. The guidelines not only take account of the level of activity which population studies suggest is protective, but also of the level and type of activity which is sustainable and can reasonably be expected of the majority of people.

Physical activity promotion in primary care

In the UK, primary care has been targeted as a major point of delivery for health promotion messages, based on the view that the physician is a powerful source of health advice. Accordingly, the promotion of physical activity in primary care has become an important issue, and the 'prescription' of physical activity by primary care physicians is currently popular. Within such schemes, physicians typically delegate the task of education and counselling in physical activity to practice nurses, or alternatively, patients are referred to physical activity 'specialists' in external venues, for example leisure centres. Exercise 'prescriptions' are often facility-based programmes, but occasionally will incorporate self-managed, lifestyle activities. Referral can be for treatment purposes, where patients may be suffering from a chronic condition known to benefit from activity (obesity, diabetes, coronary heart disease), or for preventive purposes, where currently sedentary individuals, or individuals with other CHD risk factors, are referred.

In contrast to the large number of UK schemes, evidence relating to effectiveness is sparse, and this is a matter of some concern at a time of scarce primary care resources and within a climate of evidence-based medicine. Despite the large number of schemes, the concept is still relatively new, and it is therefore unsurprising that previous reviews have identified very small numbers of published evaluations, none of which have been performed in the UK. However, one review has retrieved studies of activity promotion in a variety of settings and located over 100 papers encompassing a variety of research designs (Dishman and Buckworth, 1996).

Conclusions and implications which relate to UK policy in this field are therefore difficult to ascertain from existing reviews, as the published studies of effectiveness have taken place in the primary care systems of other countries, and have involved participants from other cultures. Further, as noted by previous reviewers, there is considerable heterogeneity in size, stated aims, type of activity prescribed, theoretical derivation, and choice of outcome measures. Findings are therefore diverse.

It has been suggested that policy in health promotion should follow careful research (ICRF Oxcheck study group, 1994), but the imbalance between the number of schemes and the lack of proven effectiveness indicates that this is not the case with physical activity 'prescription' programmes. The wisdom of introducing such programmes within primary care has therefore been challenged (Iliffe et al., 1994). Nevertheless, the continued enthusiasm for such schemes is obvious, despite the evidence from large randomised controlled trials of more general health promotion initiatives, which indicate limited effectiveness

(Family Heart Study Group, 1994; ICRF Oxcheck study group, 1994; ICRF Oxcheck study group, 1995). It is a main aim of this project to investigate this anomaly.

Evaluation of health promotion interventions

Green (1979) has suggested that three levels of evaluation are appropriate within health promotion – process, impact and outcome. Within these, various levels of design can be considered – historical record keeping, inventories, comparative and quasi-experimental, controlled experimental, evaluative. Green suggests that only the last three designs are sufficiently rigorous for health promotion evaluations. Although these suggestions are not of recent origin, this is still a sound rationale to adopt for the consideration of health promotion evaluations. The South Thames Regional Health Authority (1994) have suggested that evaluation of health promotion can be loosely classified into the categories *outcome*, *process* and *impact*, although within each of these there are problems of definition, measurement and appropriateness.

Studies which assess biological or physiological outcomes may be important in clinical terms, but are of limited use in assessing the effectiveness of health promotion schemes, because changes in these parameters tell us little about behaviour change. Further, a range of confounding factors causes difficulties of experimental control. For example diet, smoking and drug use can all affect weight, cholesterol levels and blood pressure.

What is important within health promotion is that people are persuaded to modify their behaviour. Our research questions therefore specifically address attitudinal and behaviour change, from which a range of physiological changes, and associated health benefits, are known to result. Further, improvements in social and psychological parameters are also known to accrue. The current focus of experimental studies on physiological outcomes may be restrictive, and may ignore many other potentially healthy outcomes.

A full description of review methods is contained in Appendix A. Briefly, the review methods comprised the following.

Aims

The main aim of this review was to collect and evaluate the evidence relating to primary-care based physical activity promotion schemes within the United Kingdom. More specifically, we have tried to:

- estimate the effectiveness of schemes in terms of increasing physical activity
- assess the implications of the results for existing and future practice in this area.

Research questions

Two specific research questions were defined.

- What is the effectiveness of primary-care based physical activity promotion programmes with respect to increasing physical activity levels?
- What is the effectiveness of primary-care based physical activity promotion programmes with respect to modifying mediators of physical activity, and attitudes/intentions towards physical activity?

We also sought to compare our findings with similar schemes in other countries, most notably the United States.

Retrieval strategy and procedures

Published guidelines for conducting systematic reviews of literature were obtained (EPI-Centre, 1996; NHSS Centre for Reviews and Dissemination, 1996), and used to underpin our review strategy. A systematic search of relevant databases was conducted from their year of inception to 1998. Known authors in the field were contacted by letter asking for further data or analyses, papers 'in press' or in preparation, and for any further information which would be useful for the review. Conference papers and abstracts were used to identify potential sources of data which could subsequently be subjected to quality/validity checks. We also sought to include papers in press, papers in review, theses, official reports, and other similar sources. Scheme managers were identified from databases of primary-care based projects and asked to provide measures of effectiveness and supporting methodological details. A short questionnaire was included.

Inclusion criteria

These were established as:
- studies of adults (> 16 years)
- aim of study to improve physical activity levels, mediators of physical activity, or attitudes/intentions towards physical activity
- study initiated within a primary care setting
- physical activity or related measure was an identifiable outcome measure or research focus
- study conducted within the UK.

Assessment of quality/validity

We sought to adopt an inclusive strategy, subject to quality control criteria, which encompassed quasi-experimental, observational, qualitative, and other accepted research designs in this review. The quality of studies was independently assessed by two authors on a five-point scale.

Data extraction

Data for both validity assessment (for inclusion/exclusion) and results were extracted independently using a modified version of a published form used for extracting health promotion data (NHS Centre for Reviews and Dissemination, 1996).

Data reduction

From the initial search, 254 papers relating to some aspect of physical activity promotion in primary care were identified. These papers were collected and scrutinised. Twenty-five studies were identified as being empirical in nature, and of these twelve satisfied all five inclusion criteria for the review. Table 1 contains design details of the twelve studies, and Table 2 the main results. The heterogeneous nature of the outcome measures, assessment tools, and resulting data makes a quantitative synthesis (meta-analysis) inappropriate. The extracted data are therefore presented in tabular form and are supported by a narrative discussion.

Effectiveness of UK studies

Campbell, Browne and Waters (1985), in one of the first controlled studies of physical activity promotion, studied the effects of an exercise promotion scheme in a New Forest village. The scheme was a community-based project initiated by the local GP – a well-known figure in the community. This study compares the activity levels of a random sample of the community with a random sample from a similar, neighbouring village which acted as a control. Serial measurements were also taken from both villages one year later. Activity levels were assessed by a non-validated series of questions regarding walking, more vigorous activities, and other active pursuits. The authors conclude that there were significant increases in activity levels in the intervention village during the year.

Gibbins, Riley and Brimble (1993) used a questionnaire to assess changes in perceptions, behaviours and clinical measurements in men attending well-person clinics over 3–5 years. During the initial clinics activity levels were noted, but no further details of method or validity are given. No control group was used. Upon recall, participants were asked to indicate whether their activity patterns had changed and in what direction. The authors report no changes in activity levels, although no statistics are reported.

The ICRF Oxcheck study (1994; 1995) was a large multi-site randomised controlled trial which focused upon reducing CVD and cancer risk factors via health checks conducted by nurses.

Table 1. Design details of UK studies assessing the effectiveness of primary-care based physical activity promotion schemes

Study	Aim	Inclusion criteria	Type of study	Setting	Type of intervention	Length of follow-up
Taylor, Doust and Webborn (1998)	To examine the effects of a GP exercise referral programme on modifiable CHD risk factors	Patients aged 40–70 yrs, identified as smokers, hypertensive (at least 140/90 mm Hg) or overweight (BMI > 25)	RCT	Facility-based	*Experimental group*: 20 exercise sessions over 10 wks at a leisure centre. *Control group*: No exercise sessions, no specific advice on lifestyle change. Both groups were given a leaflet on CHD risk and exercise. Measurements taken at baseline 8, 16, 26, and 37 wks	37 wks
Naylor *et al.* (in press)	To examine the effectiveness of SOC-based counselling for exercise delivered by practice nurses in 4 primary care centres	Patients attending health checks	Controlled trial	Home-based	*Experimental group*: Condition A: Stage of Change materials and counselling; Condition B: Stage of Change materials only; Condition C: Non Stage of Change based activity advice. *Control group*: Normal activity advice. Measures taken at baseline, 8 wks & 24 wks	24 wks
Stevens *et al.* (forthcoming)	To assess the cost-effectiveness of a primary-care based intervention aimed at increasing levels of activity	Inactive people aged 45–74 yrs	RCT	Facility- and home-based	*Experimental group*: personalised 10-wk programme to increase PA, combining leisure centre and home-based activities. *Control group*: information on leisure centres. Measurements at baseline and at 8-months follow-up	8 months
Riddoch *et al.* (forthcoming)	To assess the effectiveness of PA promotion interventions in a primary care setting	No specific inclusion criteria were established (as the Stage of Change model is applicable to all individuals)	Controlled trial	Home-based	*Experimental group*: Condition A: Stage of Change based leaflets and counselling; Condition B: Stage of Change based leaflets only. *Control group*: Normal activity advice Measurements taken at baseline, 8 wks and 26 wks	26 wks

Table 1. Design details of UK studies assessing the effectiveness of primary-care based physical activity promotion schemes (continued)

Study	Aim	Inclusion criteria	Type of study	Setting	Type of intervention	Length of follow-up
Munro (1997)	To evaluate an 'exercise on prescription' GP scheme	People over 65 yrs and the least active 80% in the intervention population	RCT	Facility-based	*Intervention group*: Least active patients identified and invited to attend exercise classes at a leisure centre for 2 yrs. *Control group*: Patients not invited to exercise classes. Measurements at baseline and at 10 months. Qualitative research	1 yr
ICRF Oxcheck Study Group (1995)	To determine the effectiveness of health checks, performed by nurses in primary care, in reducing CVD risk factors and cancer	Men and women aged 35–64 yrs identified from the Bedfordshire Family Practitioner Committee's register	RCT	Urban general practices	*Experimental group*: Health check in 1989–90 and a second health check 3 yrs later. *Control group*: Health check in 1992–3. Measurements taken at yr 1 and yr 4 of the study	5 yrs
Lord and Green (1995)	To evaluate patterns of compliance and changes in physical and mental health in the Stockport 'exercise on prescription' scheme	Adults 18–65 yrs not participating in regular exercise, with no contra-indications for exercise, and not at risk of CVD	Pre-test – post-test	Facility-based	*Study group*: Patients filled in questionnaires at baseline, 10 wks and 6 months. Focus groups and interviews with participants and GPs	10 wks
Vernon (1994)	To assess the effects of a GP-referral scheme on self-reported exercise levels. Stage of Change for exercise and self-efficacy for exercise	Men and women aged 16–75 yrs with low exercise levels, plus one other CHD risk factor	Controlled trial	Facility-based	*Study group*: Instructor-led sessions and self-managed activities. Minimum of 2 sessions/wk. *Control group*: Normal exercise advice	8 wks
ICRF Oxcheck Study Group (1994)	As above	As above	As above	Urban general practices	*Experimental group*: Primary health check and health counselling (15 mins) in 1989–90 and in 1990–1. *Control group*: Primary health check in 1990–1. Followed up 1 yr later	1 yr

Table 1. Design details of UK studies assessing the effectiveness of primary-care based physical activity promotion schemes (continued)

Study	Aim	Inclusion criteria	Type of study	Setting	Type of intervention	Length of follow-up
Cupples and McKnight (1994)	To assess the value of health education for patients with angina in reducing risk factors for CVD and lessening the effect of angina on everyday activities	Patients under 75 yrs who had angina for at least 6 months and did not have any other severe illness	RCT	General practices	*Experimental group:* Advice on CVD risk factors, and were reviewed and given health education every 4 months. *Control group:* Only filled questionnaires. Measurements taken at baseline and 2 yrs. Exercise levels defined as number of episodes/wk > 20 mins	2 yrs
Gibbins, Riley and Brimble (1993)	To assess the effectiveness of a programme for reducing CVD risk in men – clinical measurements and perceptions of patients	Men aged 28–60 yrs	Pre-test – post-test (no controls)	Well-person clinics in rural general practice	*Experimental group:* Health check and lifestyle counselling (10 mins). Actively intervened only for high blood pressure and high cholesterol (*N* = 136). All participants reviewed 3–5 yrs later	5 yrs
Campbell, Browne and Waters (1985)	To evaluate a health promotion campaign run by a general practitioner	The whole village of Brockenhurst	Controlled trial	Community-based	*Intervention village* (Brockenhurst): Exercise campaign initiated by GP. *Control village* (Sway): No campaign. Measurements taken before (1983) and after (1984) the exercise campaign	1 yr

Table 2. Summary of main results of UK studies assessing the effectiveness of primary-care based physical activity promotion schemes

Study	Sample size and attrition	Main outcome measures	Measurement tool for PA or associated measures	Main result	Quality score (1 = very poor, 5 = excellent)
Taylor, Doust and Webborn (1998)	345 invited 240 responded 142 randomised 41 completed study (40 intervention, 31 control)	BP, BMI, skinfold measures, smoking, physical activity	Questionnaire	87% of referees used the prescription and 28% were high adherers (15 sessions at least). Non-smokers and obese patients attended more prescribed sessions than smokers and non-overweight patients. Exercise group increased significantly energy expenditure at 8 and 16 wks ($p = 0.01$ and $p = 0.08$, respectively). Exercise group did significantly more moderate activity up to 8 wks ($p = 0.02$) and more vigorous activity up to 16 wks ($p = 0.03$). Between baseline and 26 wks, 15% more referred patients did more activity/wk than the control group. However, the difference was not significant. No change in PA was evident at 37 wks	3
Naylor et al. (in press)	294 subjects enrolled, 180 returned questionnaire at 2-months follow-up	Physical activity, Stage of Change for exercise, self-efficacy	Questionnaire	No significant differences in any measures of PA in any treatment condition across time. Significant improvements in SOC for exercise at 8 and 24 wks for the SOC materials + counselling group ($p = 0.0006$) No significant differences in self-efficacy over time for any groups	3
Stevens et al. (forthcoming)	714 (363 intervention, 351 control)	Physical activity	Questionnaire	11.2% of intervention group increased activity at 8 months compared to 0.8% in control group. Int. group reported an increase in the mean number of episodes of PA/wk (5.95 v. 4.43 $p < 0.001$)	3
Riddoch et al. (forthcoming)	406 (226 at 8-wk follow-up; 116 at 26-wk follow-up)	Physical activity, Stage of Change for exercise	Questionnaire	No significant improvement in PA. All 3 conditions – significant improvements in Stage of Change for exercise at 8 wks ($p = 0.004$)	3
Munro (1997)	9988 at baseline. Least active ($n = 2307$) invited to attend classes; 530 attended at least 1 class	Physical activity, general health status, physiological measurements, barriers, participation	Questionnaires, interviews	Participation rate 23%. 1 in 4 inactive older people may attend exercise lessons. Participation showed little fall with increasing age, with between 20 to 30% of women attending at least 1 class. Participation rates higher among women than men. Mean number of classes for men and women 25 in 10 months	2

Table 2. Summary of main results of UK studies assessing the effectiveness of primary-care based physical activity promotion schemes (continued)

Study	Sample size and attrition	Main outcome measures	Measurement tool for PA or associated measures	Main result	Quality score
ICRF Oxcheck Study Group (1995)	2205 intervention, 1916 control	Cholesterol, BP, BMI, smoking, diet, alcohol, exercise	Questionnaire	Proportion of patients reporting taking vigorous exercise less than once a month was significantly lower in the int. group (difference 3.3%) (0.5–6.1 CI)	4
Lord and Green (1995)	419 prescribed exercise, 252 attended initial consultation, 77 responded at 10 wks, 64 responded at 6 months	General health status, perceived health status, mental health status, satisfaction with the scheme, attitudes to exercise, compliance	Questionnaire	14% of those initially referred were exercising at 6 wks. 60% attended initial consultation. 18.4% compliance at 10 wks, 15.3% compliance at 6 months. Drop-out rate between 10 wks and 6 months was marginal (3%)	2
Vernon (1994)	29 intervention, 55 control; 86% response rate for experimental group, 53% for control	Stage of Change for exercise, self-reported exercise levels, self-efficacy for exercise	Questionnaire	Significant increases in Stage of Change in exp. group. No significant change in activity level in either group. No increase in self-efficacy	2
ICRF Oxcheck Study Group (1994)	2136 intervention, 3988 control	Cholesterol, BP, BMI, smoking, diet, alcohol, exercise	Questionnaire	Proportion of patients reporting taking vigorous exercise less than once a month was significantly lower in the int. group (difference 5.1%, 2.7–7.6 CI)	4
Cupples and McKnight (1994)	317 intervention, 300 control	BP, BMI, cholesterol, restriction of everyday activities, diet, smoking, exercise	Questionnaire	After 2 yrs, 44% of intervention and 4% of control groups took exercise > 7/wk, $p < 0.0001$ for trend. More of intervention group increased PA and fewer reported reduced PA than controls ($p < 0.0001$). 34% intervention and 21% control increased PA; 38% intervention and 25% control unchanged PA; 28% intervention and 54% control reduced PA	2
Gibbins, Riley and Brimble (1993)	687 males (384 seen for initial and final reviews)	Cholesterol, BP, diet, smoking, alcohol, exercise	Questionnaire	409/520 (79%) – no change in exercise 62/520 (12%) increased exercise 49/520 (9%) decreased exercise	2
Campbell, Browne and Waters (1985)	Inhabitants of Brockenhurst	Exercise	Questionnaire	Highly significant increase ($p < 0.001$) in all forms of exercise was shown in Brockenhurst when compared with Sway	1

The study reported follow-up data at 1 year and 3 years. Although the main focus was physiological risk factors, behavioural changes were reported, including physical activity. The measure of activity was in reality a measure of sedentary living, a dichotomous variable – 'vigorous exercise less than once a month'. After 1 year a 5.1% difference in activity level was observed in favour of the intervention group. After 3 years, this figure had fallen to 3.3%. At both the 1-year and 5-year follow-up measurements, results were better for men than for women. No details of the activity measure are reported nor any validity data.

Lord and Green (1995) provided a programme of three activity sessions per week of up to 1 hour's duration for a period of 10 weeks. No control group was used and activity levels were not assessed. However, the authors report an attrition rate of 82% at 10 weeks and 85% at 6 months. Forty per cent of participants failed to register for the programme, and 42% registered but dropped out. It is interesting to note that the participation rate at the end of this programme had fallen to levels similar to those normally seen in the English population as a whole (Health Education Authority and Sports Council, 1992).

Cupples and McKnight (1994) used personal health education sessions with angina patients and reported a significant trend towards more frequent exercise in the intervention group and fewer participants reducing exercise. The study used self-reported frequency of 20-minute exercise sessions – reported during interview – as the measure of activity, but no validity details are given.

Vernon (1994) achieved an 86% adherence rate in her trial, but reported no detectable improvements in activity level despite regular attendance at the activity sessions. The control group was also unchanged. This seems illogical and raises the possibilities that participants were reducing activities outside of the classes, or that the self-report method of assessing activity levels could not detect the additional activity. Increases in Stage of Change for exercise were observed in the intervention group, but no increases in self-efficacy for exercise.

Munro (1997) reports data for the first 10 months of a randomised controlled trial in Sheffield. Participants identified as 'low active' were invited to attend a 2-year programme of exercise classes. Self-reported activity levels were assessed but no data are reported. However, attendance data are reported. Of 2307 people invited to attend the classes, 15–20% attended, although this figure was improved by follow-up letters. In the first 10 months of the trial, the participation rate was 23%, with participation being defined as at least one session in the 10 months. However, this is a level of activity which will have no impact upon health. It is also reported that the most active people at baseline were most likely to attend the classes. Even within the low number of attendees, the mean number of sessions attended is 25 in 10 months – an average of approximately one session per fortnight – which is again insufficient to improve health.

The studies of Naylor *et al.* (in press) and Riddoch *et al.* (forthcoming) were replicate studies conducted in Yate and Swindon. Each study was a non-randomised controlled trial, using Stage of Change for exercise and physical activity levels as the main outcomes. Each study compared Stage of Change-based interventions, with and without individual counselling, with a non-Stage of Change-based intervention. Each study reported significant improvements in Stage of Change for the stage-based interventions, although no increases in activity levels were observed in any group. These studies used a minimal level of intervention – deemed to be deliverable within the confines of primary care resources – and a 26-week follow-up. Despite the high levels of attrition, intention-to-treat analyses showed a long-term persistence of effect on Stage of Change after this minimal and cost-effective intervention. An 8-week interim analysis showed stronger effects. These two studies were research studies only, that is they were set up specifically to assess effectiveness of nurse-administered exercise counselling. They are not continuing schemes.

Stevens *et al.* (forthcoming), in a randomised controlled trial, intervened for 10 weeks and attempted to modify activity patterns via either facility-based (leisure centre) or home-based activities. High levels of attrition were evident, but intention-to-treat analysis indicated that after 8 months 11% of participants in the intervention group increased their activity levels versus 1% in the control group. A validated self-report activity assessment method was used.

Taylor, Doust and Webborn (1998) offered a programme consisting of 20 cut-price leisure-centre based exercise sessions over a period of 10 weeks. The activity comprised moderate to vigorous aerobic activity in a semi-supervised environment. From initial referral, 87% of participants used the programme, but only 28% completed at least 15 sessions. As measured by self-report questionnaire, significantly higher levels of moderate activity were observed in the intervention group at 8 weeks, and higher levels of vigorous activity were seen at 16 weeks. No differences between intervention and control groups were seen at 26 weeks.

It should be remembered that not all of the above studies had physical activity as the main outcome measure. In many studies, activity was one of a range of outcomes, and, more importantly, some interventions were not specifically designed to increase activity levels. Interventions were often multifactorial, including dietary and smoking advice, and many included physiological risk measurements (for example blood pressure, cholesterol) as additional outcomes. In such circumstances, any observed changes in activity levels would be encouraging.

In summary, the majority of studies report some form of improvement in either physical activity or related measures. However, the size of the effect is generally small, and there is no real consistency across studies. Not all of the above studies are true 'exercise on prescription' schemes, where physical activity was the main, or the sole, outcome measure. In those studies which are, there are indications that small but possibly significant improvements in activity or activity-related measures are identifiable.

Effectiveness of non-UK studies

Eight studies met the main inclusion criteria, but are non-UK based. The main results of these studies are contained in Tables 3 and 4.

It can be seen from Table 4 that the general pattern of results is towards a small but significant improvement in activity behaviour as a result of physical activity promotion. However, follow-up periods are short, and the scale of improvement is small. Nevertheless, there is sufficient evidence to suggest that these schemes do have a limited effect. It is of interest to note that the PACE (Physician assisted Assessment and Counselling for Exercise) study (Calfas et al., 1996), which measures activity levels with an objective method (Caltrac™ accelerometer), has the most encouraging results, possibly highlighting the importance of using a sensitive activity monitoring instrument.

The PACE study is also striking in that it targets participants in an appropriate state of readiness to change (the 'contemplation' stage in the Stage of Change model). The PACE study is therefore a clear example of a primary-care based study where the intervention is soundly based in relevant theory and assessment of main outcomes is by sensitive, pre-validated objective methods.

The other striking feature of the non-UK studies is the lack of involvement of leisure centres. Interventions rely upon personal contact, mailshots and counselling procedures, without referral to external venues and external activity specialists. This is a striking and major difference in the philosophy of exercise programming on the two sides of the Atlantic.

In summary, the effects observed in these studies are of the same limited nature, but in the same positive direction as the UK studies.

Table 3. Design details of non-UK studies assessing the effectiveness of primary-care based physical activity promotion schemes

Study	Country	Aim	Inclusion criteria	Type of study	Setting	Type of intervention	Length of follow-up
Swinburn et al. (1998)	New Zealand	To find out whether written advice from a general practitioner increases PA more than verbal advice alone	Inactive patients who were likely to benefit from an increase in PA	Randomised controlled trial	Home-based	*Intervention group:* Condition A: Written exercise prescription. Condition B: Verbal advice only. Measurements taken at baseline and 6 wks	6 wks
Calfas et al. (1997)	USA	To determine to what extent: (a) a stage-matched PA intervention produces changes in mediators drawn from social-cognitive theory and the Transtheoretical Model, (b) mediators explain changes in PA	At least 18 yrs of age, sedentary, apparently healthy, and to have a scheduled 'well office' visit in the next 3 to 6 wks	Controlled trial	Home-based	*Experimental group:* Patients received physician PA counselling (3 to 5 mins) + mailed postcard as a prompt and phone conversation 2 wks later. *Control group:* Patients received no PA counselling. Outcomes measured at baseline and at 4 to 6 wks	6 wks
Marcus et al. (1997)	USA	To test the feasibility and efficacy of a physician-delivered physical activity counselling intervention	Patients who were 50 yrs or older, able to speak and read English, active less than 3 times/wk for 20 mins each time, and able to walk unassisted	Sequential comparison group design	Home-based	*Experimental group:* Exercise counselling (3 to 5 mins) + self-help materials. *Control group:* Normal care. Measurements at baseline and 6 wks after office visit for both groups. Both groups received phone calls 2 wks after initial visit. Experimental group also received phone-call follow-up at 4 wks after the initial visit	6 wks control measures, plus 6 wks intervention measures
Wiesemann et al. (1997)	Germany	To evaluate: (a) Can a GP health programme reduce behaviour-related CVD risk factors? (b) Can exercise-based groups lead to motivation for changing unhealthy behaviour?	Population of the German CINDI area over the age of 16	Repeated survey on random sample	Facility- and home-based	One study group formed by 3 levels: 1. Individual health advice given to patients by GPs 2. Group education programmes given to patients based in exercise by GPs 3. Exercise-based group education programmes given to patients by GPs. Cross-sectional data taken from 7 practices at 1992, 1993, 1994 and 1995	4 yrs

Table 3. Design details of non-UK studies assessing the effectiveness of primary-care based physical activity promotion schemes (continued)

Study	Country	Aim	Inclusion criteria	Type of study	Setting	Type of intervention	Length of follow-up
Calfas et al. (1996)	USA	To examine the efficacy of a physician-based counselling programme to promote adoption of regular physical activity by sedentary adults	Sedentary patients over age 18, free of CHD or other conditions that limit mobility, who were scheduled for a 'well office' in the next 3–6 wks	Controlled trial	Home-based	*Experimental study group:* Patients received physician PA counselling (3 to 5 mins) + brief booster phone call 2 wks after. *Control study group:* Patients didn't receive PA counselling. Measurements taken at baseline and at 4–6 wks follow-up in both groups	6 wks
Burton et al. (1995)	USA	To test the impact of physician visits as a method of encouraging health behaviour change among community-dwelling older persons	65 years old and over, with a primary care physician who was participating in the study	Randomised controlled trial	Home-based	*Experimental group:* Patients offered 2 preventive examinations and optional counselling visits for 2 years (1 examination each year). *Control group:* Normal care	2 yrs
Graham-Clarke and Oldenburg (1994)	Australia	To evaluate the effectiveness of an exercise intervention developed for use by general practitioners with patients	Patients from both sexes, aged 18–69 years, who were found to have one or more modifiable CVD risk factors	Randomised controlled trial	Home-based	*Study group A:* Routine care. *Study group B:* Lifestyle counselling using videos. *Study group C:* Lifestyle counselling using videos and self-instructional materials. Assessments conducted at baseline. after 4–6 months and at 12–18 months	2 yrs
Lewis and Lynch (1993)	USA	To examine the impact of brief exercise advice-giving by family physicians	Outpatients aged 18 and older who were scheduled to see a doctor	Controlled trial	Home-based	*Phase 1:* Patients were queried about their exercise habits and attitudes, and whether their physician had discussed exercise. *Phase 2.* *Experimental group:* Administered brief exercise protocol (2 to 3 mins) by physicians. 2 subgroups in experimental group – prompted and unprompted. *Control group:* Normal care. Measurements taken at baseline and 1 month	4 months

Table 4. Summary of main results of non-UK studies assessing the effectiveness of primary-care based physical activity promotion schemes

Study	Sample size and attrition	Main outcome measures	Measurement tool for PA or associated measures	Main result
Swinburn et al. (1998)	239 'green prescription' group (218 completed) 252 verbal advice group (238 completed)	Physical activity	Questionnaire	Percentage of people engaging in any PA increased from 54% to 81% in both groups. Number of individuals participating in any PA from baseline to follow-up: follow-up was significantly greater in the exercise prescription group ($p = 0.004$). Number of participants that increased the total amount of PA was higher in the prescription group ($p = 0.02$). Substantial increases in duration of PA were seen in both groups but were not statistically significant ($p = 0.16$). Self-reported PA increased from 36% to 68% in the prescription group. This was a greater increase ($p = 0.02$) than for the verbal advice group (40% to 57%). 43% subjects in the prescription group reported an increase in their PA over the previous 2 months, as opposed to 37% in the verbal advice group ($p = 0.10$)
Calfas et al. (1997)	98 intervention group, 114 control group	Physical activity. Stage of Change for exercise. Processes of change. Self-efficacy. Social support	Questionnaire, accelerometer and walking habits	Patients who were counselled improved significantly more than those in the cont. group on behavioural and cognitive processes of change ($p < 0.001$, $p < 0.05$, respectively). Other changes in mediators were non-significant. Psychosocial mediators accounted for 11% of the variance in walking score. Psychosocial mediators accounted for 9% of the variance in the Stage of Change score. Self-efficacy accounted for 10% of the variance in change in accelerometer score
Marcus et al. (1997)	63 patients agreed to participate in the study. 44 completed the study (19 intervention, 25 control)	Physical activity. Stage of Change for exercise	Telephone interviews, questionnaire	PA scores remained unchanged in controls. PA scores increased from a mean of 148 to a mean of 154 in experimental group. Multivariate results revealed a 17.6-point difference (effect size 0.20) in PA scores for experimental patients compared with controls ($t = 1.32$, $p = 0.19$)

Table 4. Summary of main results of non-UK studies assessing the effectiveness of primary-care based physical activity promotion schemes *(continued)*

Study	Sample size and attrition	Main outcome measures	Measurement tool for PA or associated measures	Main result
Wiesemann et al. (1997)	3485 subjects participated out of 4881 examinations. 600 subjects were included in exercise-based groups out of 1347 examinations	CVD risk factors, smoking, habitual exercise, engagement in sports, complaints of the joints, dietary habits, stress levels, nicotine consumption and drugs, importance of health	Questionnaire	73.5% repeated increased activity levels. Only 18.3% of drop-outs reported relapse into sedentary behaviour
Calfas et al. (1996)	98 intervention group. 114 control group	Physical activity. Stage of Change for exercise	Questionnaire, accelerometer and walking habits	Experimental group reported increased walking more than cont. (+37 min/wk v. +7 min/wk). ($p < 0.05$). Experimental group 33% increase in PA when measured by accelerometer ($p < 0.005$). Controls showed a decrease in PA. Self-reported PA measurement was non-significant. At follow-up, 52% int. adopted regular activity (moved from contemplation to action), compared with 12% of cont. ($p < 0.005$)
Burton et al. (1995)	3097 interviews obtained (1573 intervention, 1524 control)	Smoking. Problem alcohol use. Sedentary lifestyle. Health status	Questionnaire	No difference between the exp. and cont. groups in the proportion with improvement in sedentary lifestyle. Being in the intervention group did not increase the odds ratios significantly for sedentary lifestyle
Graham-Clarke and Oldenburg (1994)	80 general practitioners and 758 patients	Physical activity. Intention to change	Questionnaire	Increase in energy expenditure over the 12 months ($p = 0.0001$) although the difference between groups was not significant. After adjusting for age, sex and Stage of Change for exercise, there was a significant increase in energy expenditure over the 12 months ($p = 0.0001$). 22% of patients showed positive progression in Stage of Change for exercise in the intervention group at 4 months, and 21% at 12 months. However, this difference is not significant
Lewis and Lynch (1993)	211 participants	Exercise duration and frequency	Interviews	Among patients receiving advice, there were statistically significant increases in minutes of exercise/session and minutes of exercise/wk ($p < 0.01$), but not in the number of times patients exercised each week. Prompted and unprompted advice resulted in significant increases in mins/wk exercise ($p < 0.04$, $p < 0.02$, respectively). Those receiving unprompted advice exercised significantly more mins/session ($p < 0.02$). Patients receiving advice were more likely to participate in any form of exercise ($p = 0.04$) and to participate in a second form of exercise ($p = 0.03$)

Grey literature

Forty-five questionnaires and supporting documentation were received from scheme managers, comprising project reports, results of evaluations, completed questionnaires, and personal observations and information. Much of this material has been gathered for internal purposes, and demonstrates that evaluation is perceived as an important aspect of this dimension of health promotion.

Only three schemes (7%) carried no reference to evaluation. However, as the initial request was for data relating to evaluation, it is likely that schemes that were not conducting evaluations did not respond. Forty-one schemes (93%) were either in the process of putting evaluations in place, or were currently conducting some sort of evaluation. Of the 41 schemes involved in evaluation, 30 (73%) were assessing physical activity levels, 9 (22%) programme adherence, 17 (41%) mediators of activity (for example self-efficacy, Stage of Change for exercise), 14 (34%) cost-effectiveness, and 36 (88%) other health benefits (for example weight, blood pressure). Only three schemes reported the use of recognised research tools (SF-36, Allied Dunbar Fitness Scale). In the great majority of cases, where the research design and analytical procedures are reported, they are seriously flawed, thus limiting the level of interpretation which can be placed on the data. Many schemes report that no data are yet available.

The general impression gained from scrutiny of the internal evaluations is that the results are generally more favourable than the published studies. In other words, one gets a more positive feeling of effectiveness reading these evaluations compared to reading the published reports. Some of the reported effects are extremely large. However, design weaknesses may be a cause of this, as poor designs are known to give more optimistic results in intervention trials. There is also a tendency to over-generalise findings, selectively report positive findings and to discuss the data without reference to the methodological limitations. Despite the relatively large volume of data emanating from unpublished sources, and its more positive findings, it would be unwise to base future policy on such data, as they are almost universally flawed in scientific terms.

Biddle, Fox and Edmunds (1994) concluded in their review that no examples of good evaluation were found, and Fox *et al.* (1997) have suggested that this is due to a lack of resources. We believe that the situation is now improved, and have identified a small number of promising examples of internal evaluations, often by individuals who are using the study as a dissertation project within a higher degree programme. However, none met the criteria for inclusion in the review. We have also been informed of planned evaluations which also have input from research organisations, principally universities. One gets the feeling that if these efforts could be harnessed into a co-ordinated, more rigorous framework, then a large quantity of valid data could be easily accumulated. The Health Education Authority (1996) have issued guidelines on evaluation, which could form the basis of such a venture.

It is interesting to note that few schemes reported the use of a psychological model of behaviour change, and that in no case were details available. This may be a major factor limiting the effectiveness of schemes.

Main aim

To assess the wider impact of exercise on prescription schemes additional to physical activity effects on patients.

Objectives

- To identify elements which are perceived to contribute significantly to the success of schemes.
- To explore the variety of effects that exercise prescription schemes have on all involved, in addition to the referred patients.

Selection of schemes

We sought to identify schemes which covered a variety of designs and modes of delivery. The following range of factors was considered:

- length of time in existence
- scale of operation
- adherence rates
- achievement of goals
- theoretical basis
- involvement of local authority
- physical activity message promoted
- facility- or non-facility based
- ability to accommodate the research within the timescale of the project.

Participants

We intended to obtain data from:

- general practitioners
- practice nurses
- exercise specialists

- health authority/health promotion specialists
- other staff involved in the scheme, including receptionists (of both GPs and leisure centres) and liaison officers
- partners, family and friends.

For confidentiality and ethical reasons no data were collected from patients.

Techniques

Three case studies were conducted, to incorporate varied geographical location, range of activity 'prescriptions' and messages, different settings for activity, and involvement of local authorities. Data collection was carried out over 3–4 days within each location, and included semi-structured interviews, informal discussions, job shadowing, document searches and observational techniques. The focus of the case studies was on the perceptions of effectiveness and the overall level of impact, beyond the specific effects on referred patients. Included in this were potential effects on scheme administrators, doctors, nurses, leisure centre staff and families of patients. A list of topical questions used in these studies is contained in Appendix B.

Semi-structured interviews were used. Issue-oriented questions were listed that were read to each respondent during individual sessions. The interview was piloted before being used. Note-taking and immediate post-session writing up of data were carried out. During observation sessions, efforts were made to minimise influence on what was taking place.

Data analysis

Data were analysed by searching for patterns and consistencies within response categories. Differences and similarities between the patterns identified in each case study were then sought in order to provide an overview. A list of potential response categories is contained in Appendix B.

Location and organisation

This scheme is located in a small town within a mainly rural county in the south-west of England. The scheme was formally established in May 1996. A healthy community forum provided funds for the initial start-up costs, which included production of a patient leaflet and laminated information cards for use in primary care. No funding was made available for the continuing management of the project and it is reliant on the provision of a reduced pricing policy by the leisure providers (£2.50/session) and supervision by health promotion services.

The organisations involved in the scheme are two private leisure centres, one local authority leisure centre, 14 general practices, and the health authority. The scheme is based on both facility- and home-based exercise programmes. Hence, there are three different methods of referral.

- 'Personal Action Plan': involves setting targets in the home environment to increase physical activity (for example housework, gardening).
- 'Doorstep walks': referral to a package of walks around the town; patients can participate in these walks either on their own or as an exercise session from one of the leisure centres.
- 'Prescription for Activity' scheme: referral to leisure centres.

Data sources

The sources of information used to assess the perceived impact and success of the scheme are based on a document search, observation and semi-structured interviews with the health promotion officer, exercise instructors and practice nurses.

Impact of the scheme

- An evaluation report of the first 6 months did not show any significant increase in physical activity at work, at home, for transport or in spare time, despite an increased frequency of moderate activity found immediately after the 12-week programme. However, the overall consensus of people involved in the scheme is that it is very successful. The scheme is seen as having a wide range of positive effects, mostly of a personal and social nature.

- The scheme is perceived as giving patients the chance to meet people who have experienced a similar illness, or similar experiences in life, and therefore they receive support and encouragement from each other. New friends are made, and social interaction is encouraged through participation in organised events (for example Christmas lunch, talks about health-related issues, going for coffee after walking or exercising). Patients feel they belong to a group and to an organisation, and the psychological benefits they receive from this are perceived as very important.

- The scheme allows relationships between patients and leisure centre staff to develop, sometimes to the extent that a genuine friendship is developed. Leisure centre staff report that they receive a greater sense of achievement from referred patients than from more typical leisure centre visitors.

- Patients were thought to have become less depressed, anxious and stressed, and also to have improved their self-esteem. Self-confidence is developed. As a consequence, patients' outlook on life might change, becoming more positive. If patients have gone through a serious illness or surgery the scheme might afford them a chance to become more independent, more functional and able to regain their former lives.

- Exercise is seen as one of the few, if not the only, things that can have so many different positive effects on different types of people, different types of health problems and within different personal situations.

- The community benefits in that a 'snowball' effect is thought to occur. Friends, partners and family are encouraged to join the scheme or to exercise.

- General practitioners and practice nurses reported increased awareness of the positive changes that regular exercise can produce. Doctors, some of whom were initially quite sceptical about exercise, have adopted more positive attitudes towards exercise. Doctors were surprised at the observed level of benefit in patients. Some practice nurses have joined the scheme. One practice nurse explained that she now visits the leisure centre regularly, and that this is immensely valuable as it is the only time she has for herself, and she insists that everybody respects it. Since she joined the scheme, she explained that her husband and some friends have also joined – as a result of her improved looks and healthier/fitter disposition.

Primary care staff perceive that encouraging patients to exercise can make their job easier, as some patients will not need to visit the doctor as often.

Being involved in the scheme has also affected the way practice nurses talk about lifestyle to the patients. They now understand that it is not just a matter of giving leaflets to patients, but there is a need to *show* them what they can do to improve their health. In this way, nurses are encouraging patients to take more responsibility for their own health.

Perceptions of success

Factors identified as positively contributing to the success of the scheme included enthusiasm, choice between facility-based and home-based programmes, good communication between leisure centres and general practices, confidence in exercise specialists, clear referral procedures, monitoring of patients' progress, individual prescriptions and supervision, and enjoyment.

Location and organisation

This scheme is located in a large town on the outskirts of one of north-west England's largest cities. The scheme is a partnership between the health commission, an NHS healthcare trust and leisure services. The scheme received its first referrals in October 1992 and more than 2000 people have been referred since then. The scheme has a relatively high budget which is received from the local authority, the city council and various local grants.

The scheme is community-based, using a wide range of leisure centres throughout the town. The centres offer a variety of supporting facilities, for example crèche facilities, and a free mini-bus to take people to the swimming-pool. Leisure centres are situated within a variety of socio-demographic areas, enabling patients to select one in which they will feel comfortable. There is a wide range of activities, catering for all patients' needs. A 'football on prescription' scheme and an obesity programme are also offered, and home-based programmes are available when the more formal activities are not suitable for patients. Patients pay £5.65 for 40 exercise sessions. Patients are given information about exercise and can always contact the exercise officer whenever necessary.

Data sources

Data were obtained from shadowing the exercise officer in whatever he was doing. So, information was taken mostly from observation and informal discussions with practice nurses, exercise instructors and the exercise officer.

Impact of the scheme

- Internal monitoring indicates that upon completion of the scheme only a minority continue attending exercise classes. The main reason for this is that participants have to start paying for the exercise sessions. As many people using the scheme are low-income, this is a major issue.
- Patients suffering from stress, anxiety, depression and loneliness are observed to change their outlook on life as a result of participating in

this scheme. These patients do not only get the benefits of exercise but the benefits of a better social life, meeting new friends, feeling 'looked after' and supported by staff and other patients.

- Some patients without health problems feel the need to see the doctor and request something to make them 'feel better'. Joining the scheme is seen as providing a positive contribution to health and reduces anxiety.
- Patients are perceived to gain knowledge concerning their own health and fitness, and the scheme is therefore seen to play an important role in preventive medicine.
- Exercise is thought to improve patients' self-esteem and self-confidence, and these improvements change the patients' perception of life – even to the extent that their life might be revolutionised.
- Improvements in psychological health are expected to reduce other health-damaging behaviours such as smoking and poor diets.
- Some physical health problems are perceived to disappear through exercise when the origin of the problem is psychosomatic.
- The scheme is seen as being a 'meaningful' factor in many patients' lives. Such positive personal changes are reported to have a continuing effect within the family environment.
- Additional recruitment to the scheme has been reported as a result of observing marked changes in the appearance and demeanour of patients.
- The scheme is seen as important because it operates in areas of the city where crime rates are high, and physical activity is seen as a possible way of moderating this.
- Leisure centre staff enjoy helping people solve both their mental and physical problems. Furthermore, the staff feel they are providing a valuable and important service to the community as they give the chance of exercising to people who would have never done it otherwise.
- It is rewarding if patients are seen to use the information and knowledge given.
- The scheme takes pressure from doctors, as everybody attending the surgery can be offered 'something' which will benefit them in some way. This is particularly important for those people who do not feel well, but in whom no illness can be detected.
- Doctors feel a reduced pressure because patients now have an exercise specialist to talk to about health-related issues, thus reducing their work burden.
- Practice nurses and doctors report that their views about exercise have changed since they have been involved with the scheme. At the beginning they felt that the scheme was only for 'sporty' people or athletic people who wanted to get fit. Now, they realise that anybody can experience the various health benefits of exercise, particularly those people with psychological problems.
- Primary care staff have realised that the scheme helps patients to take

responsibility for their own health. Consequently, they feel that it is an excellent way to save money in the long term, although for GPs this is very difficult to quantify.

- The scheme has made GPs aware that prescribing exercise is not as simple as it seems, and that qualified exercise specialists are needed to work in this field.
- From a personal point of view, the scheme has made doctors realise that they should do more exercise themselves, in order to get the same benefits that they see in patients. They also report a more positive attitude towards preventive medicine.
- Practice nurses also explained that there is a different reaction to the scheme between the sexes. Women are more sensitive, functional and more interested in health than men and therefore they react very positively to the scheme. In contrast, it is more difficult for men to join the scheme as it means they have to accept there is something wrong with them.
- The fact that women join the scheme is perceived to have an impact on their husbands, as they feel pressure to join the scheme as well.

Perceptions of success

Factors identified as positively contributing to the success of the scheme included enthusiasm, availability of the exercise specialist, individual programming and support, talking and listening to patients, dealing with patients as people – not diseases, the low cost, variety of activities, variety of locations, independence of patients during exercise sessions, and promotion by the media.

Location and organisation

This scheme is located near the centre of one of north-west England's largest cities. The scheme is facility-based, with eight leisure centres and over 50 GPs referring patients. The scheme has been running for nearly four years, with more than 900 patients referred since January 1996. The scheme is an initiative of the a local community trust (NHS) and the city council leisure services in conjunction with the health authority. The scheme is seen as an important element of the strategy to achieve the physical activity targets stated in the City Health Plan.

The scheme is leisure centre-based, and offers a variety of activities at low cost. Each leisure centre offers a specific timetable for referrals, and because eight leisure centres are involved in the scheme the timetable covers the whole week. Patients can therefore exercise every day if they wish. Patients have the chance to join a Fit for Life programme when they finish participating in the initial scheme, and there is an exercise programme for ethnic minorities.

Data sources

The data from this case study have been taken from documents, observation, semi-structured interviews and informal discussions with health promotion officers, leisure centre managers, exercise instructors, and practice nurses.

Impact of the scheme

- The scheme is perceived to have a wide range of effects on all involved in it. The scheme helps patients to combat loneliness, to meet new friends, to receive support from others who are in the same position, to feel a sense of identity with a group of people, and to feel 'looked after'. Self-esteem and self-confidence are thought to be improved.
- Referred patients are perceived as 'non-sporty' people who enjoy talking, laughing and sharing stories with others, as well as exercising.

- Patients share the common purpose of becoming healthy and fully able to enjoy life, and the 'group effort' is perceived as important, especially for older patients.
- The scheme provides support, and opportunities for experience-sharing and making social contacts.
- Patients who have a family history of ill health often report that they are concerned about the future. The scheme gives these people the opportunity to do something positive about their health, and about their future.
- For older people, the scheme enables them to feel that they are taking steps to counteract the inevitable effects of the aging process. It gives them the feeling that they are doing something positive with their lives.
- Exercise is perceived to become a main priority in the lives of a significant number of patients.
- Participation in the scheme is perceived to improve functionality and quality of life – particularly the ability to cope with the activities of daily living.
- For some individuals the scheme has been instrumental in getting them out of the house on a regular basis.
- The scheme is perceived as being suitable for 100% of the population, because exercise is the only 'prescription' which meets many needs with many answers.
- Organisers of the scheme are aware that 'proving' effectiveness is problematical. In particular, an assessment of how *significant* the scheme becomes in many people's lives needs to be assessed. Tying shoelaces for the first time in many years can have a major impact upon life, but will be missed by most physical activity assessment techniques.
- The effectiveness of the scheme is considered to relate more to how membership of the scheme affects people's quality of life and happiness, rather than in quantifying how much additional exercise they take. If patients feel better, more independent and more self-confident, the scheme is successful.
- Some people who would have never attended a leisure centre are now doing so because of the scheme. This is perceived as very beneficial for the leisure centres, as patients sell and promote the centre to other people. Thus, a message is transmitted that leisure centres are not only for 'sporty' people but also for everyone who wants to exercise.
- Some leisure centres were grant-aided to purchase new equipment to guarantee the quality of the scheme, and the scheme is perceived to have attracted new and 'different' types of instructors to the leisure centres.
- Instructors have adapted and expanded their knowledge and adapted their philosophy of exercise.
- Instructors are now more aware of how intimidating they can be to many referred patients who actually fear exercise.

- Overtly 'healthy' people – both instructors and leisure centre users – develop a greater awareness of the sort of health problems that some people have. Being involved in the scheme has raised the instructors' level of job satisfaction.
- The workload within the general practices is perceived to be reduced, as patients can now talk to the instructors about their health concerns, rather than the doctor or nurse.
- Patients who just feel 'unwell', but for whom no illness can be detected, are often referred to the scheme and there is a perception that they visit the doctor less frequently as a direct result.
- The scheme is perceived as being very effective in treating people suffering from depression. The scheme acts as a reason for depressed patients to get out of bed and out of the house. The effects of the scheme in this situation are perceived to be immediate, and therefore very valuable.
- Doctors are keen that they now have an alternative, non-pharmacological treatment to offer certain patients instead of drugs.
- Patients perceive a better 'service' because they are offered a course of treatment that is supervised and tailored to each patient's needs. Some patients have changed their general practice because their original practice was not referring patients to the scheme.
- Primary care staff are enthusiastic about the scheme because it helps to demonstrate their commitment to health promotion. The promotion of physical activity could not be used in such an effective way without membership of this scheme.
- Some primary care staff have joined the scheme as they get a free pass from the leisure centres. As a result they become familiar with the experiences of patients on the scheme and also act as an example for patients who are uncertain about joining the scheme. As a result, exercise has achieved a higher profile within primary care, as doctors and nurses have been able to experience and understand the benefits of exercise for both treating and preventing illnesses.
- In some practices, joining the scheme was perceived as adding extra work to their normal duties. However, this was slowly replaced by an understanding that workloads might eventually be reduced, supplemented by a real appreciation of the potential benefits to the patients. An investment of time and patience is perceived to be needed at the outset in order to acquire the long-term benefits.

Perceptions of success

Factors identified as positively contributing to the success of the scheme included a high perceived need within the community, enthusiasm, partnership between leisure centres, primary care, the health authority and the health promotion services, supportive GPs, low-cost alternatives, easy access to leisure centres, flexibility of activities, exercise programmes for cardiac rehabilitation patients and ethnic minorities, clear referral procedures, supervision and monitoring by exercise specialists, a supportive environment – not 'sporty', and promotion by the media.

Experimental studies

The results of the review can be viewed as encouraging, in that improvements in physical activity and associated measures are evident in many studies. It is clear that well-planned programmes can have significant effects on physical activity behaviour and on psychological and health-related factors which are related to physical activity. The majority of well-conceived studies do show a positive effect, but the size of effect diminishes with increasing rigour of study design. No studies demonstrate a negative effect, with the exception of the adherence data, which is disappointing across nearly all studies. The remarkably high attrition rates noted in many studies is a matter of considerable concern.

Biddle, Fox and Edmunds (1994) concluded that the schemes which they studied were successful, in that they were popular with patients, physicians and leisure centre staff, but that no rigorous evaluation of effectiveness could be identified. The situation now is that the number of schemes has proliferated, the majority are still seen as successful, and that there are emerging indications of success in terms of their primary aims – the improvement of activity behaviour.

We are particularly aware of one very important limiting factor. Subtle changes in certain dimensions of physical activity are known to be beneficial to health. However, appropriate health-related dimensions of activity are often not included in evaluations, and also the methodologies used to measure activity are normally crude and unable to identify such changes. There is a high probability that small but important changes are missed by current evaluation procedures.

One further major limiting factor is the lack of long-term follow-up of participants. Whereas a 10-week study can be sufficient to demonstrate *efficacy*, i.e. that a programme is able to modify behaviour in ideal circumstances (for example for the duration of a programme), a longer-term study is required to demonstrate *effectiveness*, i.e. the level of success achieved among all those to whom it is offered (post-programme adherence). In other words, the level of *adherence* to the programme must be included. It is in the field of effectiveness where the UK data are currently weak.

We are aware of the current scarcity of published data in this relatively new field, and that much of the data we have reported accrue from small-scale pilot studies. Nevertheless, despite the lack of large-scale randomised controlled trials focusing specifically on modifying physical activity behaviour, we believe that these studies are of sufficient quality to provide a sound body of evidence from which tentative conclusions can be drawn. Interestingly, in a meta-analysis of over 100 physical activity promotion interventions, Dishman and Buckworth (1996) found no differences between the results of quasi-experimental studies and randomised controlled trials. It is nevertheless prudent to discuss only the general pattern of results in this review, rather than the size of effect. At this stage we are merely trying to ascertain the existence and direction of an effect, rather than the effect size.

Our conclusions relating to the UK data are in agreement with reviews of non-UK randomised controlled trials, both in the size and direction of effect. However, it is clear that whereas the overall picture is positive, not all studies demonstrate an effect; but whether lack of observed effect is due to measurement deficiencies or lack of statistical power cannot be ascertained.

In order to appreciate the true value of these schemes, a number of factors need to be considered. We have observed a consistent pattern of improvement in activity behaviour, and this must be considered against the size of effect which interventions of this nature might be expected to have. All health-related behaviours are notoriously stable, and it is our view that the indications of effectiveness seen here are indeed meaningful. It is unrealistic, and theoretically unsustainable, to expect substantial improvements in activity levels in large numbers of people. Other behavioural interventions, for example smoking cessation and weight loss programmes, can also have small but meaningful effects if well designed.

Physical activity is a complex behaviour, and the danger of adopting unrealistic expectations must be avoided (Godin and Shephard, 1983). The level of effect seen in these studies can be compared favourably to the results of studies adopting a population approach. For example, Tudor-Smith et al. (1998) have reported that activity levels in Wales increased significantly during the five years of the Heartbeat Wales programme. However, similar increases in activity were observed in a reference area with no intervention.

It is interesting to note that when the results of two large-scale, multifactorial health promotion interventions (Family Heart Study Group, 1994; ICRF Oxcheck study group, 1994) were reported, the small but significant effects were reported in terms of general failure. This demonstrates an over-optimistic perception of realistic and achievable effects, and also reflects an interpretation of results from an individual perspective from what were essentially minimal interventions, conducted within a large population of participants. From a population perspective, the results of these studies could be considered surprisingly positive, given the limited strength and the nature of the interventions. In a similar vein, Iliffe *et al.* (1994) have warned against the adoption of activity promotion schemes in the absence of evidence of effectiveness. They identify a variety of uncertainties which might be susceptible to research, and many of these are as yet unresolved. It is interesting to note that schemes continue to proliferate, suggesting that even in the relative absence of effectiveness data, schemes are perceived as successful at least in the terms adopted by those professionally involved.

As mentioned previously, there are two competing factors on the level of effect. Firstly, there is a high potential for measurement error in the assessment of physical activity, and this will result in an overly pessimistic outcome. Subtle changes in behaviour cannot be detected by the crude measures of activity normally obtained, and this will serve to dilute the intervention effect. On the other hand, quasi-experimental designs, the majority in this review, are known to produce overly optimistic results. These two factors may serve to balance each other out, but the relative strengths of each are impossible to ascertain.

The difficulties of improving activity levels should not be underestimated. The very low adherence rates seen in these studies is testament to this. Studies in which the design and delivery of programmes are more firmly rooted in physiological and psychological theory – in particular where an accepted model of behaviour change is used – undoubtedly demonstrate better results. Appropriate targeting of participants by psychological readiness to change, as evidenced by the PACE study (Calfas *et al.*, 1996) in the US, is also more effective. Failure to target effectively will undoubtedly result in low uptake and adherence rates, and can be considered a substantial wastage of resource. As early as 1983 Godin and Shephard realised the naiveté of not adopting a tested method of behaviour modification, and yet the great majority of schemes still do not incorporate this as a design feature.

It should also be considered that carefully constructed experimental studies, designed to identify a single behavioural modification in a single group of participants, cannot assess the true impact, in the widest sense, of the intervention. Ebrahim and Davey-Smith (1997) have argued that randomised controlled trials are more appropriate for high-risk participants than for population and social approaches to prevention. Similarly, Redman (1996) has argued that some health promotion programmes may have 'failed' because they focus on individuals, rather than environmental issues. For example, the narrow focus of a randomised controlled trial will miss the potential effects on physicians, nurses, ancillary staff, exercise referral staff, leisure centre staff, health promotion specialists, and the family and friends of the participants who are studied.

Case studies

All three schemes are considered very successful, being different in location (for example rural versus urban), and setting (for example leisure and home based, community based and leisure-centre based).

Of particular note is the common factor between all schemes – that a wide range of impact is perceived, involving many individuals other than the patients. Whereas the effects on patients may be seen as treatment, the effects upon other individuals may be fulfilling a preventive role.

Further, it should be noted that the impact upon the patients is consistently perceived to be at the social and psychological levels – whereas schemes are normally set up to impact upon physiological factors, for example the classical CHD risk factors. The reasons for this discrepancy between original intentions and retrospective evaluations of impact are worthy of further consideration.

It is also clear from these studies that all of these schemes are perceived to have similar effects. In particular, the benefits of just being a member of a scheme appears important, as this has a wide range of effects on social and psychological factors. Membership has an important impact on the patients' lives, and even small achievements can be meaningful. Patients find support, a social life, and self-confidence. They might be happier and experience an improved quality of life. Exercise has become recognised as possibly the only means of producing a large variety of meaningful effects on a variety of people.

It is also clear that the schemes are seen to be particularly effective with certain types of patients. In particular, patients suffering from anxiety or depression are seen to benefit greatly. Also, patients who report feeling unwell, but in whom no illness can be detected, also seem to benefit. It may be the case that for these patients non-pharmacological treatment is particularly appropriate, and that exercise might distract their attention, or give the patients a new focus. It also possible, of course, that schemes are used by doctors as a means of relieving the frequency and the stress of dealing with some difficult-to-treat patients. It is clear that individualised prescriptions and supervision are important factors, particularly for patients who are initially fearful of exercise.

There are, however, perceived weaknesses. Firstly, the fixed length of programmes means that effects are normally short term, unless a continuing strategy is available for patients at the end of the programme. Secondly, evaluation is a problem, in that the diverse range of effects, and the various types of people who feel effects, are difficult to assess, particularly in the absence of funding and training in evaluation techniques. The profit motive of the leisure centres is seen as a problem, although there are also signs that leisure centres do adopt a positive and non-profit approach to the schemes.

It is possible to identify four common factors which consistently appear to contribute to the success of these schemes: staff enthusiasm; working within alliances and maintaining good communications between the organisations; designing individual exercise programmes tailored to each patient's needs and having individual supervision; and having a low-cost policy, especially in areas of low income.

Summary

The results of the two stages of this review are complementary, in that the experimental data suggest small, positive effects, and the case studies suggest wider-ranging and more significant effects. Taken together, we consider that the evidence is generally positive. However, it should be considered that the evidence is also limited in both scope and volume, and that further research is undoubtedly necessary. In particular, research that adopts design features which can assess the total impact of schemes is encouraged.

It is of particular note that the observed effects are seen in schemes which are generally not based on a sound theoretical model. Further, the common choice of leisure-centre based activity sessions may also be counter-productive for many individuals, and this strategy may need further consideration. It may be that home-based activities, use of community settings and family-based activities may all have important roles to play in the future.

Our general impression is that the growth and development of schemes has been dramatic, but the level of theoretical input has been low. If this were to be introduced, then schemes could expand into new areas, and incorporate a wider variety of settings, more flexible prescriptions, improved support strategies for patients and long-term provision of low-cost support structures when patients leave the scheme. If standardised procedures for accurate data gathering could also be introduced and co-ordinated, then more accurate measures of impact and effectiveness could be obtained on a regular basis.

10. Conclusions and recommendations

Systematic review

A careful consideration of the accumulating evidence leads to the tentative conclusion that primary-care based physical activity promotion schemes have small but positive effects on some participants. There are a number of encouraging factors. Firstly, given the considerable methodological limitations and complexities of defining and assessing physical activity behaviour, the detection of positive changes is a considerable achievement. Secondly, the majority of studies reviewed used cost-effective interventions which are feasible within the budgetary confines of the primary care setting. Thirdly, improvements in Stage of Change for exercise have been observed at 26 weeks after an intervention which comprised just one counselling session (Naylor *et al.*, in press). Fourthly, there is obviously a considerable enthusiasm for such schemes, both within primary care, health authorities and leisure services, and the large scale of operation which now exists will have a considerable impact within a more global physical activity promotion campaign.

There are, nevertheless, a number of aspects which deserve further consideration. Firstly, there is a distinct lack of contemporary theoretical input to the design and delivery of the great majority of schemes. Secondly, the choice of leisure centres as the setting for activity can be problematical for many individuals. Thirdly, the quality of most internal evaluations is poor, and therefore a great opportunity to assess wide-scale effectiveness is currently being missed.

The findings can be summarised as follows.

- The studies reviewed here demonstrate small but possibly meaningful improvements to physical activity patterns and other activity-related measures.

- As far as we can detect, no existing UK programmes are based on an accepted model of behaviour change. This is an area where considerable further input at both design and delivery stages is needed.

- The activity message delivered is often based on a fitness training model which is now considered inappropriate, if not counter-productive.

- The leisure centre setting may be inappropriate for some people. The reasons for referring to leisure centres may be rooted in a fitness training/sport perception of health-related activity, which is inappropriate. Alternative venues may need to be considered.

- More flexibility of activity prescription is necessary to take account of psychological readiness to change, participants' personal goals, current activity status, and health status.

- Appropriate professional training must be developed for physical activity referral specialists in the health field. Most exercise specialists have qualified in sports science, where the body of knowledge, although related, is in many ways insufficient to deal effectively and safely with all participants. In particular it is important that exercise specialists are educated in what constitutes safe and effective exercise for individuals who vary markedly in age, health status, level of motivation and goals. No longer are they dealing predominantly with young, fit individuals. The use of accepted motivational strategies and psychological models of behaviour change will also be important.

- There is a lack of quality evaluations of physical activity promotion schemes in the UK. Whereas rigorous evaluation via large randomised controlled trials is only possible with substantial research grants, it should nevertheless be possible to monitor the effects on participants in a more systematic way. Simple designs and cost-effective data-gathering procedures should be possible. Such a surveillance system would provide strong evidence which can inform policy. There is also a need for training in evaluation procedures for relevant staff.

- Appropriate criteria for referral to an activity programme should be developed, to take account of health status, activity status and motivation to change. Activity programmes should also be seen as a preventive strategy as well as a curative strategy.

- Expectations of programme success should be realistic. Major changes in large numbers of participants will not happen, as can be seen in smoking cessation and weight loss initiatives. Small effect sizes are encouraging, not problematic.

- Supporting environmental initiatives may need to accompany activity promotion programmes. Intentions and attempts to change stand less chance of success if the local environment is not supportive of health-related activities.

Case studies

The data from the three case studies tell a completely different story to the data from the systematic review. From the case study data it is apparent that the schemes are perceived to have considerable impact not only upon the patients, but also on primary care staff, leisure centre staff, communities, and friends and colleagues of all involved. Membership of a scheme *per se* is seen as contributing beneficially, for a variety of reasons. This leads to the realisation that studies of effectiveness are likely to miss many real effects of a scheme, as they focus upon physical activity levels, often measured by inaccurate methods which fail to pick up subtle changes in behaviour.

Likewise, the effects on patients are diverse, and sometimes surprising, given the original aims of many schemes. It is particularly noticeable that whereas many schemes include a variety of physiological measurements as part of their evaluation procedures, the main effects on patients are in the social and psychological domains. Whereas schemes are seemingly set up to affect, for example, blood pressure and weight, the actual effects are in different areas. This has implications for the type and nature of evaluation procedures which scheme managers might incorporate.

The findings can be summarised as follows.

- The effects of schemes are seen to have an impact not only upon patients, but on many other people who are directly and indirectly associated with the schemes.
- The effects are seen in a wide variety of social and psychological parameters which are not easily evaluated.
- Certain types of patient are seen to benefit particularly, for example patients with psychological disorders, or those patients in whom illness cannot be detected.
- The existence of schemes has done much to promote the status of physical activity as a health-related issue and to dispel its 'sporty' image.
- Many people associated with schemes have changed their views about what constitutes health-related physical activity, and have modified their approach accordingly.
- There is a consistent range of process factors which contribute to success. However, there is no 'blueprint' for success.

11. Implications for design and evaluation

Many factors can influence the actual and assessed level of effectiveness of a scheme. Such factors can relate to the design and delivery of the programme itself – in other words well-designed programmes are likely to have a greater beneficial effect. Also, research design factors can determine whether the true effects of the programme are isolated and accurately quantified. The more important influencing factors should be considered by both programme designers and researchers, and some of these are discussed below.

Programme factors

Promotion of appropriate activity messages

Guidelines for a healthy level of activity focus upon the equivalent of 30 minutes' brisk walking on most days of the week (Department of Health, 1996). One of the main factors underpinning this message is that this type and level of activity is more achievable and sustainable than fitness-related activity 'messages' which focus upon a minimum of three sessions of at least 20 minutes of vigorous activity per week. The brisk walking message is also more appropriate for individuals of advancing years and for individuals with chronic conditions. It is therefore interesting to note that relatively few schemes incorporate the 'newer' message. The majority of schemes focus upon facility-based programmes, although home-based or lifestyle-based activities are sometimes offered as an additional option.

Selection of appropriate activity settings

As previously mentioned, many UK schemes focus upon group or class activities, performed in a leisure setting, for example a local sports centre. However, it is not clear that the literature supports this strategy, especially in terms of uptake and adherence to programmes. For example, walking is often reported to be a highly popular activity (Booth *et al.*, 1997) and it is clear that this activity does not require attendance at a class or the existence of a group. However, supervision and the security of having an 'expert' on hand was identified in the case studies as being an important motivating factor for some patients. Godin and Shephard (1983) have noted that the majority of physical activity interventions are targeted at the most affluent members of society. Whether this is the case in the UK is difficult to ascertain, but it is an important aspect in the light of current public health policy (Department of Health, 1998), which highlights the importance of 'hard-to-reach groups'.

In this respect it is interesting to note that although activity promotion is initiated within primary care, the setting for the activity intervention is often a leisure centre, which may not carry appropriate connotations for large sections of society. In the Yate 'Get Moving' study Naylor *et al.* (1998) offered a reduced rate leisure centre pass as part of their intervention, but only 1% of participants took advantage of it. Stevens *et al.* (1998) have reported that the proportion of sedentary participants using leisure centres increased from 4% to 16% during their intervention. The authors also report that all participants were active away from the leisure centre at least as often as within it. Webborn (1996) has reported that only 20% of leisure centre referral patients continued to use a leisure centre on completion of the programme. On the other hand, Gould, Iliffe and Thorogood (1997) have reported mixed views among physicians about the appropriateness of primary care as a health promotion setting, and they state that the suitability of primary care as a setting is as yet unresolved.

There is an interesting comparison to be drawn between the UK and the US data. In contrast to the UK systems, US projects focus more upon lifestyle activity and home-based activity. This may be a contributory factor in the slightly more positive results seen in the US studies. It may be that a more appropriate setting is one based in the community, but which does not carry sporting connotations – for example the proposed healthy living centres.

Individual prescriptions

It is important that programmes have systems to ensure that people and prescriptions are matched carefully. For many participants, an activity programme will be inappropriate in the first instance, until the individual feels more at ease with the concept of becoming more active. Prescription of a standard activity programme for all referred participants is to be avoided for safety, effectiveness and motivational reasons. This practice ignores the fact that different activity programmes can stimulate different physiological responses. More importantly, there is abundant evidence that only a minority of people are psychologically 'ready' to become more physically active. For such individuals, the delivery of an action-oriented prescription (an activity programme) will be counter-productive. Targeting by current activity status may be more productive, possibly facilitated by using the Stage of Change model, as reported in the PACE programme (Calfas *et al.*, 1996).

Selection criteria for referral

Effectiveness will be reduced if inappropriate people are referred. It is clear that the great majority of schemes adopt a 'treatment' perspective, rather than a 'prevention' perspective, as indicated by the common practice of targeting people who have pre-existing disease. Many schemes target people with CVD risk factors, which may be considered a preventive strategy, but relatively few schemes target currently healthy, but sedentary, people. It may be argued that primary care does not have the resources, and is not the appropriate setting for such a 'population' strategy. As pointed out by previous authors (Ashenden, Silagy and Weler, 1997; Ebrahim and Davey-Smith, 1997) a treatment perspective, targeting the fewer people who have chronic diseases known to be susceptible to physical activity, may be more in line with the physician's traditional role. In this way it might also be argued that more effort can be concentrated on fewer people, thus maximising chances of success.

Kreuter *et al.* (1997) in a survey of 915 adults and 27 physicians, have reported that physicians are most likely to provide physical activity advice to patients who are already sick (especially overweight). Neither current activity levels nor readiness to change was related to the type of patient referred. The authors suggest that physician behaviour in this respect may systematically exclude patients who may be most appropriate for intervention.

Delivery of programmes

It is generally accepted that education alone, or the giving of activity advice, is ineffective in stimulating behaviour change. However, strategies for delivering programmes effectively do exist, including negotiation, identification of Stage of Change, delivering stage-matched messages, and motivational interviewing (Rollnick, Kinnersley and Stott, 1993). In this respect, the qualifications of referral specialists, whether they are practice nurses or leisure centre staff, are of prime importance. Exercise specialists require specialist training, and this is not included in the typical sports science degree. Participants in activity referral schemes are often at the opposite end of the activity and motivational spectrum, and often have chronic disease. Such individuals demand a completely different approach to the young, healthy athlete who is training for performance. A high level of professional training is required in this specialist area.

Use of appropriate delivery strategies

The design and delivery of schemes have a critical impact on effectiveness. Dunn (1996) has indicated that we are beginning to develop the tools and strategies necessary to intervene in the high-risk behaviour of physical inactivity. Particularly in the US, programmes and research efforts have broadened from rigidly defined exercise sessions in supervised gym-based programmes to include many other, more moderate intensity, activities in more naturalistic settings. However, it is a general criticism of UK schemes that although some take account of such developments, the great majority do not. Some schemes are now incorporating the 'moderate' message, but many still rely on cardiovascular fitness principles.

The great majority of schemes are class-based and facility-based – mostly in leisure centres, and very few schemes use a discernible model of behaviour change. Dunn (1996) has further suggested that home-based programmes based on shorter bouts of activity may play an important role in the adoption of physical activity, and it is clear that the great majority of UK schemes do not take account of this. Many, indeed, do the opposite. These factors may not be unrelated to the high levels of attrition commonly reported in UK schemes.

Powell *et al.* (1991) have suggested that health promotion applies a variety of strategies (for example information dissemination, skill building), in a variety of settings (for example worksite, school), to a variety of target groups (for example children, elderly). They suggest that achieving the optimum match of elements from each dimension maximises effectiveness. Other theoretical perspectives on health promotion are available, for example the Precede–Proceed model (Green and Kreuter, 1991). The Transtheoretical model (Prochaska and DiClemente, 1983) has been successful in modifying other behaviours and has been adapted for physical activity (Marcus *et al.*, 1992). Materials based on this model are available through the Helping People Change programme and the guidance booklet *Promoting physical activity through primary health care* (Health Education Authority, 1996).

However, in the UK no schemes responding to this study report that they use such a strategy and the great majority appear to be atheoretical in their approach to changing behaviour. It appears that the 'cart has come a little before the horse', in that the rapid expansion of the number and scale of schemes has far outstripped the level of theoretical input which they have been given. It may be appropriate at this stage to take stock of the current situation and ensure that the design, delivery and evaluation of schemes are firmly based within the best evidence available. It may also be prudent to consider whether supporting educational and environmental initiatives may further enhance effectiveness.

Provision of supportive environments

Godin and Shephard (1983) have suggested that asking people to alter their lifestyles will not work if the environment is not supportive of such changes. The promotion of activity in the absence of a supportive environment may therefore severely limit effectiveness. Environmental influences can be family support (verbal, practical, participative), safe activity locations (for example well-lit walking/jogging trails, existence of cycle paths), or extrinsic motivational techniques (for example mileage allowance for cycling to work, or provision of showers and safe cycle storage facilities in the workplace).

Research design factors

Choice of research design

Virtually all the published literature is experimental. Whereas such methods are undoubtedly important, as they isolate the primary outcome measure – the physical activity of participants, they give no information regarding the wider impact of a programme, for example the effects on participants other than the referred patients. Many schemes have attracted wide media attention, potentially raising awareness of the health benefits of physical activity in the community. Leisure centre staff might adopt a broader view of health-related physical activity and motivational factors as a result of dealing with 'patients' rather than athletes. It is interesting to speculate that possibly unintended effects on staff may enhance programme delivery, as regularly active practice nurses have been shown to be more likely to promote activity than irregularly active nurses (McDowell, McKenna and Naylor, 1997).

A pluralistic approach to the evaluation of health promotion interventions (Beattie, 1995; Bowler and Gooding, 1995) might provide a more accurate estimation of the true *impact* of the intervention, in its widest sense, still recognising the importance of the primary outcome – the specific effects on participants. It may be that a case study approach to evaluation might be at least as rewarding as a randomised controlled trial. With the exception of the three case studies incorporated in this review, we can identify no other studies which have adopted this approach to assessing the overall impact of schemes.

Selection of appropriate outcome measures

Authors of the influential ICRF Oxcheck study used physiological variables as their main outcome measures, whereas the Yate 'Get Moving' researchers chose Stage of Change for exercise as the main outcome. Each of these is indicative of different underlying views of what constitutes a realistic and meaningful effect. It might be argued that without physiological changes health will not improve, but, as argued previously, the physiological mechanisms via which activity improves health are largely unknown, making the selection of appropriate and meaningful physiological outcome measures difficult.

In terms of effectiveness, the true outcome of an intervention aimed at improving activity levels is physical activity itself, and it is probably more prudent and meaningful to assess activity, as indicated by the strong epidemiological evidence suggesting a positive reduced risk with increasing levels of activity. However, it has been hypothesised that large numbers of people are not prepared to consider increased activity, and that for them it is unrealistic to expect behaviour change. Attitudes and intentions towards activity can be modified, however, and these can serve as appropriate outcomes in physical activity promotion studies. By doing this each participant has the potential to improve, not just the few who are 'ready' to take up activity.

As previously discussed, the wider impact of schemes is almost universally ignored in the published literature. As evidenced by the results of our case studies, this may be a major and misleading omission.

Accuracy of measurement

The importance of accurate assessment of physical activity and its associated measures has been acknowledged in one review (Dishman and Buckworth, 1996). Mostly it is ignored. This is surprising, as physical activity is the main outcome measure under review and is notoriously difficult to measure. It is a complex and infinitely variable behaviour with many dimensions. Further, there are controversial conceptual issues about which is the most appropriate health-related dimension of physical activity, and this is also seldom addressed. Both the accuracy of measurement and the selection of an appropriate activity dimension will have a major impact upon results and their interpretation.

Objective methods (motion sensors, heart rate monitors, observation) carry the highest validity, but are time-consuming and expensive. They are therefore not normally considered feasible for anything but small studies. Self-report measures are notoriously inaccurate, and even with the compensation of large numbers, and the associated statistical power, such inaccuracy is problematical. This is a more serious problem than is normally realised. Firstly, many self-report measures of activity assess inappropriate dimensions of activity. For example, it is common to assess sport or vigorous leisure-time activities. In both of these cases other non-sports or non-vigorous activities are ignored. Secondly, many self-report methods are gender-biased, in that they ignore home-based activities, many of which are still performed predominantly by women. Thirdly, the measurement error inherent in self-report methods are considerable and can be of greater magnitude than the subtle differences in activity which interventions might be expected to achieve. The risk of type II errors (failing to detect a real effect) is therefore substantial.

It is interesting to note that in the PACE study (Calfas et al., 1996) activity levels assessed by self-report methods showed no significant changes, whereas the *same* activity measured by motion sensors (Caltrac™ accelerometers) showed significant changes. In the interests of obtaining valid activity data, it is strongly recommended that in future studies objective measures of activity are used. The cost and logistical implications of this are obvious, but only by such methods can subtle modifications to activity behaviour be detected.

Length of follow-up

The health benefits of activity are transient, and therefore nothing less than long-term effects are meaningful. Whereas referral schemes commonly involve activity programmes of a number of weeks, participants are often left to their own devices at the end of the programme. From a public health perspective, it is what happens after the programme is finished which has the most impact upon health. Very few studies assess this, and extremely few internal evaluations address the problem. Whereas it might be a simple task to assess adherence and activity levels during the programme, especially if it is facility based, it is far more problematical – but far more important – to evaluate events during the post-programme period.

Godin and Shephard (1983) have suggested that short-term effects may not translate into long-term gains, and that few benefits persist more than 1–2 years. The same authors also discuss the possibility of a 'halo' effect, or 'Hawthorne effect', whereby early improvements are not only related to the nature of the intervention, but also to the process of 'being studied'. In fact Green (1979) has described health education as no more than an 'organised placebo'. While this may be a radical view, it is clear that adequate control of such factors, through long-term follow-up, is therefore of great importance.

Inappropriate analyses

The *efficacy* of physical activity is well established, in that it is known to modify a variety of health-related physiological and psychological parameters. In this review, we have looked at studies which address the *effectiveness* of variety of procedures to promote behaviour (physical activity) change. A basic principle in the assessment of effectiveness is to include in the analysis all participants to whom the intervention was offered, irrespective of whether or not they complied fully with the programme (intention-to-treat analysis). It is noticeable that few studies analyse their data in this way, most notably the internal evaluations. This is a major limiting factor to many of the studies retrieved.

It is also common in effectiveness trials to establish a minimum effect size which is considered important and then to discuss differences between group means in relation to this effect size. If the mean difference between treatment and control is less than the smallest change which is important, then the intervention is commonly deemed to have had a minimal impact. However, by doing this the distribution of effects is ignored, and if the effects are in fact heterogeneous then a significant proportion of participants may have benefited from the intervention even though the group effect size is small.

Godin and Shephard (1983) have recognised that in physical activity intervention studies relatively few people change their behaviour, and yet comparison of group means is normally the choice statistic. They suggest that the key variable of interest is the proportion of people who comply/change in the long term. Investigators are therefore encouraged to report this type of statistic. For example, Guyatt *et al.* (1998) encourage the use of proportions of participants who improve, deteriorate or remain the same as a meaningful outcome measure. These data are more informative and give a more realistic estimation of the true impact of the intervention. It may be particularly relevant for behavioural interventions, where effects are likely to be heterogeneous, and where the outcome variable is continuous. Such an approach does not obviate the need to exclude chance factors, rather it supports the notion of conducting additional, more informative analyses.

12. Future developments – healthy living centres

The results of this review can be considered with respect to future developments in health promotion. One such development is the proposed healthy living centres (HLCs), which may have an important role to play in the future of exercise prescription schemes. HLCs will be based in the community, and run for the community. In this way, they may be seen as a welcoming environment in which to discuss health matters. Their location in 'health action zones' may enable them to attract sections of society who do not traditionally attend leisure centres or fitness clubs – where most exercise referral schemes are currently based. If these centres are to be used, it will necessitate an increased focus on lifestyle activity, or home-based activity, both of which are theoretically justified. Although some people undoubtedly enjoy attendance at a leisure centre, there are others for whom such places are forbidding, and this may indeed be linked to the high attrition rates we have observed. Although close supervision and class- or group-based activities are reported to be popular, there are nevertheless extremely high attrition rates from the majority of leisure-centre based schemes. It is interesting to note that in the USA leisure centres are not used in primary-care physical activity promotion schemes – they prefer to rely on counselling strategies and home- or lifestyle-based activities.

Because most facility-based schemes are for a fixed period, long-term continuation of facility-based exercise relies upon long-term availability of money, transport, and access to a leisure centre. Home-based exercise or lifestyle exercise does not require any of these and may be behaviourally more sustainable in the long term.

Should schemes be based in HLCs, there are implications for the approach adopted by the exercise specialist. Because traditional fitness facilities may not be generally available, a counselling approach may be needed. This will have additional implications for the level and type of training such staff receive. There is also the possibility that exercise can be dealt with in conjunction with diet, stress and smoking, in order that a more complete approach to healthy living can be adopted.

There are also ways in which facility-based schemes and HLCs can work together. As previously mentioned, the fixed length of leisure-centre based schemes poses considerable problems for patients when their programme finishes. Without an obvious choice of what to do next there is a high chance of relapse into sedentary behaviour. It is conceivable that HLCs can provide the necessary continuing support systems that are required in order to maximise the chances of permanent changes in behaviour.

HLCs could therefore provide a complementary support strategy to the work of the leisure centres, and they could also constitute a completely different strand of physical activity promotion – targeting other groups. They may also be better able to set physical activity into a more holistic lifestyle framework.

Appendix A. Systematic review – methods

Review strategy

Published guidelines for conducting systematic reviews of literature were obtained (EPI-Centre, 1996; NHS Centre for Reviews and Dissemination, 1996), and used to underpin the review strategy adopted. Our procedural aim was to minimise bias at all stages of the review, and we therefore adhered to a chronological procedure incorporating the following stages:

1. establishment of study aims
2. establishment of research questions
3. establishment of literature retrieval procedures
4. establishment of study inclusion criteria
5. establishment of quality/validity criteria
6. data extraction procedures
7. analysis.

Stages 1 and 2 were agreed by a project steering group. Stages 3–7 were conducted by the research team. All judgements relating to study inclusion, quality assessment and data interpretation were made independently by at least two authors. Results were compared, discrepancies were discussed and decisions taken.

Aims

The main aim of this review was to collect and evaluate the evidence relating to primary-care based physical activity promotion schemes within the United Kingdom. More specifically, we have tried to:

- estimate the effectiveness of schemes in terms of increasing physical activity and related parameters
- assess the implications of the results for existing and future practice in this area.

Research questions

Two specific research questions were defined.

1. What is the effectiveness of primary-care based physical activity promotion programmes with respect to increasing physical activity levels?

2. What is the effectiveness of primary-care based physical activity promotion programmes with respect to modifying mediators of physical activity, and attitudes/intentions towards physical activity?

We also sought to compare our findings with similar schemes in other countries, most notably the United States.

Retrieval strategy and procedures

A systematic search of relevant databases was conducted from their year of inception to 1998. These included MEDLINE, Embase, PsychLIT, BIDS, DARE and EPI-Centre. One internet database (Pubmed) was also searched. MEDLINE was considered to be the most lucrative source, and an optimally sensitive search strategy for health promotion (NHS Centre for Reviews and Dissemination, 1996) was adapted for this project. Specific terms entered included 'randomised controlled trial', 'exercise', 'physical activity', 'primary care', 'counselling', and 'health education'.

In all databases key terms were entered as title words and also as abstract text words. Various combinations of terms were entered. Searches were also carried out on main authors' names and 'other related articles'. Known books, book chapters, and reviews were searched manually. Reference lists of retrieved articles were also searched manually. Searches of recent editions of key journals were undertaken to identify studies not yet indexed. Known authors in the field were contacted by letter asking for further data or analyses, papers 'in press' or in preparation, and for any further information which would be useful for the review. Follow-up letters and telephone calls were made to non-responders as appropriate.

Conference papers and abstracts were used to identify potential sources of data which could subsequently be subjected to quality/validity checks. We also sought to include papers in press, papers in review, theses, official reports, and other similar sources. This 'grey literature' was subjected to identical inclusion and validity checks to the published data. Written permission was obtained to include unpublished data.

Scheme managers were identified from databases of primary-care based projects, and asked to provide measures of effectiveness and supporting methodological details. All health promotion units in England were contacted to provide further contacts with schemes.

Inclusion criteria

Inclusion criteria were established *a priori* by the review team. The lack of UK studies, and very few world-wide, indicated that broad inclusion criteria were necessary:

- studies of adults (> 16 years)
- aim of study to improve physical activity levels, mediators of physical activity, or attitudes/intentions towards physical activity
- study initiated within a primary care setting
- physical activity or related measure was an identifiable outcome measure or research focus
- study conducted within the UK.

Assessment of quality/validity

There are considerable practical and logistical difficulties in performing randomised controlled trials in primary care settings (Bowler and Gooding, 1995), and there is also some debate whether undue emphasis is placed on the randomised controlled trial in assessing effectiveness (Pringle and Churchill, 1995; Mant, Dawes and Graham-Jones, 1996; Speller, Learmonth and Harrison, 1997). Further, guidelines for conducting systematic reviews (NHS Centre for Reviews and Dissemination, 1996) do not limit reviews to RCTs, especially if this compromises the volume of material collected. The guidelines state that a variety of designs can be included as long as appropriate inferences are made, in accordance with the strength of the design. We have therefore not limited our review to randomised controlled trials. We sought to adopt an inclusive strategy, subject to quality control criteria, which encompassed quasi-experimental, observational, qualitative, and other accepted research designs in this review.

In order to maximise inclusion, trials were not rejected on grounds of limited length of follow-up, although we appreciate that long-term behaviour modification is required in order to gain health benefits. Such a procedure would have severely limited our search, and we felt it necessary to discuss effectiveness in the light of all available evidence. Further, the length of follow-up necessary for meaningful health gain to occur is unknown.

The quality of studies was assessed according to:

- design
- size and statistical power
- choice of outcome measures
- quality of measurement of outcomes
- theoretical basis of content and delivery of intervention
- quality of delivery of intervention
- length of follow-up.

The quality of physical activity assessment, and/or related parameters, was considered to be a particularly important aspect of design, as it is a major source of error often not addressed by authors or reviewers. The measurement error inherent within self-report methods of physical activity assessment is considerable, and can severely limit the significance of results. Further, because activity behaviour is resistant to change, and might be expected in only a minority of individuals, it is equally important to assess mediators of physical activity, for example attitudinal and intentional parameters which, while not being behaviours, are important steps upon the way to behaviour change. In this way, the true level of impact, across the whole study population, can be evaluated.

Studies were rated on a five-point scale according to design, size, choice of outcome measures, quality of measurement (particularly physical activity), theoretical derivation of intervention, quality of delivery of intervention and length of follow-up.

Data extraction

Data for both validity assessment (for inclusion/exclusion) and results were extracted independently using a modified version of a published form used for extracting health promotion data (NHS Centre for Reviews and Dissemination, 1996, annex I). Where discrepancies occurred, issues were discussed and resolved by the assessors. Where papers were unclear, attempts were made to contact authors for clarification. Assessors were not blinded to the authors or to the results. All relevant data were entered on to a relational database (Microsoft Access).

Appendix B. Case studies – topical questions and response categories

Topical questions

1.1. Do you think this 'exercise on prescription' scheme is successful?

1.2. Why do you think it is successful or why not?
  (a) Because of the staff working on it
  (b) Because of the materials and resources available
  (c) Because of the structure of the scheme
  (d) Because of the sequence of service provided to the participants
  (e) Because of the content of the exercise prescription/counselling
  (f) Because of the way the exercise prescription/counselling is delivered
  (g) Because of the environment that surrounds the scheme:
    (g.1) Environment with lots of people self-motivated to exercise
    (g.2) Environment with lots of inactive people
    (g.3) Environment that potentiates the practice of physical activity and exercise (for example lots of parks and walk paths)
    (g.4) Environment that supports people who are active (for example family, friends, organisations)
  (h) Others

2.1. Does the 'exercise on prescription' scheme affect you?

2.2. In which way?:
  (a) From an emotional point of view (e.g. I feel happier)
  (b) From a social point of view (e.g. I have lots of new friends)
  (c) From a cognitive point of view (e.g. I have learnt a lot about exercise and the functioning of my body)
  (d) From a health point of view (e.g. My health is much better)
  (e) From a behavioural point of view (e.g. My lifestyle is much better now)
  (f) Others

2.3. Does the 'exercise on prescription' scheme affect people around you in some of the ways mentioned above?
  (a) Partner
  (b) Family
  (c) Friends
  (d) At work
  (e) Others

2.4. Does the 'exercise on prescription' scheme affect the organisations involved?
  (a) Primary care
  (b) Leisure centre
  (c) Health authority

2.5. In which way?
  (a) Resource allocation
  (b) Scientific orientations
  (c) Economic orientations
  (d) Philosophical orientations
  (e) Political orientations
  (f) Others

Response categories

1. History/background (method: documents)

2. Process (method: interviews – documents)

General information:
  Funding
  Organisations involved
  Individuals involved
  Setting

Factors that make a programme successful:
  Staff working on it
  Materials and resources available
  Structure of the scheme
  Sequence of service provided to the participants
  Content of the exercise prescription/counselling
  Way the exercise prescription/counselling is delivered
  Environment that surrounds the scheme:
      people self-motivated to exercise
      inactive people
      that potentiates the practice of physical activity and exercise (for example parks and walk paths)
      that supports people who are active (e.g. family, friends, organisations)
  Others

3. Impact (method: interviews)

Effects of the scheme on:
    Knowledge
    Attitudes and intentions (emotional point of view)
    Behaviour change
    Perceived health status (psychological and physiological)
    Assessed health status (psychological and physiological)
    Social life
    Others
In whom?
    Patients
    General practitioners
    Practice nurses
    Fitness leaders
    Local health authority
    Other staff involved in the scheme: receptionists of both GPs and
    leisure centres, liaison officers
    Staff and patient's partners, family and friends

In which organisations?
    Primary care
    Leisure centre
    Health authority

In which way are the organisations affected?
    Resource allocation
    Scientific orientations
    Economic orientations
    Philosophical orientations
    Political orientations
    Others

Anderson, R E, Blair, S N, Cheskin, L J and Bartlett, S J (1997). Encouraging patients to become more physically active: the physician's role. *Annals of Internal Medicine.* **129**(5):395–400.

Ashenden, R, Silagy, C and Weler, D (1997). A systematic review of the effectiveness of promoting lifestyle change in general practice. *Family Practice* **14**(2):160–76.

Beattie, A (1995). Evaluation in community development for health: an opportunity for dialogue. *Health Education Journal* **54**:465–72.

Berlin, J A and Colditz, A (1990). A meta-analysis of physical activity in the prevention of coronary heart disease. *American Journal of Epidemiology* **132**:612–27.

Biddle, S, Fox, K and Edmunds, L (1994). *Physical activity promotion in primary health care in England.* London: Health Education Authority.

Blair, S N (1995). Exercise prescription for health. *Quest* **47**:338–53.

Blair, S N, Kohl III, H W, Barlow, C E, Paffenbarger, R S, Gibbons, L W and Maccra, C A (1995). Changes in physical fitness and all-cause mortality: a prospective study of healthy and unhealthy men. *Journal of the American Medical Association* **273**:1093–8.

Booth, M L, Bauman, A, Owen, N and Gore, C J (1997). Physical activity preferences, preferred sources of assistance, and perceived barriers to increased activity among physically inactive Australians. *Preventive Medicine* **26**:131–7.

Bowler, I and Gooding, S (1995). Health promotion in primary health care: the situation in England. *Patient Education and Counseling* **25**:293–9.

Britton, A, Thorogood, M, Coombes, Y and Lewando-Hundt, G (1998). Search for evidence of effective health promotion (letter). *British Medical Journal* **316**:703.

Burton, L C, Paglia, M J, German, P S, Shapiro, S and Damiano, A M (1995). The effect among older persons of a general preventive visit on three health behaviors: smoking, excessive alcohol drinking, and sedentary lifestyle. *Preventive Medicine* **24**:492–7.

Calfas, K J, Long, B J, Sallis, J F, Wooten, W J, Pratt, M and Patrick, K (1996). A controlled trial of physician counseling to promote the adoption of physical activity. *Preventive Medicine* **25**:225–33.

Calfas, K J, Sallis, J F, Oldenburg, B and French, M (1997). Mediators of change in physical activity following an intervention in primary care: PACE. *Preventive Medicine* **26**:297–304.

Campbell, M J, Browne, D and Waters, W E (1985). Can general practitioners influence exercise habits? Controlled trial. *British Medical Journal* **290**:1044–6.

Chapman, T (1996). *1996 directory of GP-referred exercise schemes in England.* Chichester: Chichester Institute of Higher Education.

Cupples, M E and McKnight, A (1994). Randomised controlled trial of health promotion in general practice for patients at high cardiovascular risk. *British Medical Journal* **309**:993–6.

DeBusk, R F, Stenestrand, U, Sheehan, M and Haskell, W L (1990). Training effects of long versus short bouts of exercise in healthy subjects. *American Journal of Cardiology* **65**:1010–13.

Department of Health (1992). *The health of the nation: a strategy for health in England*. London: HMSO.

Department of Health (1996). *Strategy statement on physical activity*. London: Department of Health.

Department of Health (1998). *Our healthier nation: a contract for health*. London: Stationery Office.

Department of Health and Human Services (1996). *Physical activity and health: a report of the Surgeon General*. Pittsburgh, PA: Department of Health and Human Services, Centers for Disease Control and Prevention, National Center for Chronic Disease Prevention and Health Promotion.

Dishman, R K and Buckworth, J (1996). Increasing physical activity: a quantitative synthesis. *Medicine and Science in Sports and Exercise* **28**(6):706–19.

Dunn, A L (1996). Getting started – a review of physical activity adoption studies. *British Journal of Sports Medicine* **30**:193–9.

Eaton, C B and Menard, L M (1998). A systematic review of physical activity promotion in primary care office settings. *British Journal of Sports Medicine* **32**:11–16.

Ebrahim, S and Davey-Smith, G (1997). Systematic review of randomised controlled trials of multiple risk factor interventions for preventing coronary heart disease. *British Medical Journal* **314**:1666–74.

EPI-Centre (1996). *EPI-centre review guidelines*. London: Social Science Research Unit, London University Institute of Education.

Family Heart Study Group (1994). Randomised controlled trial evaluating cardiovascular screening and intervention in general practice: principal results of British family heart study. *British Medical Journal* **308**:313–20.

Fletcher, G F, Blair, S N, Blumenthal, J, Caspersen, C, Chaitman, B, Epstein, S, Falls, H, Sivarajan Froelicher, E S, Froelicher, V F and Pina, I L (1992). Statement on exercise: benefits and recommendations for physical activity programs for all Americans. *Circulation* **86**(1):340–4.

Fox, K, Biddle, S, Edmunds, L, Bowler, I and Killoran, A (1997). Physical activity promotion through primary health care in England. *British Journal of General Practice* **47**:367–9.

Gibbins, R L, Riley, M and Brimble, P (1993). Effectiveness of programme for reducing cardiovasular risk for men in one general practice. *British Medical Journal* **306**:1652–6.

Godin, G and Shephard, R J (1983). Physical fitness promotion programmes: effectiveness in modifying exercise behaviour. *Canadian Journal of Applied Sport Science* **8**(2):104–13.

Gould, M M, Iliffe, S and Thorogood, M (1997). Is physical activity on the primary health care agenda? *World Review of Nutrition and Dietitics* **81**:160–6.

Graham-Clarke, P and Oldenburg, B (1994). The effectiveness of a general-practice-based physical activity intervention on patient physical activity status. *Behaviour Change* **11**(3):132–44.

Green, L W (1979). How to evaluate health promotion. *Hospitals* 1 October, pp. 106–8.

Green, L W and Kreuter, M W (1991). *Health promotion planning: an educational and environmental approach*. Palo Alto, CA: Mayfield Publishing Company.

Guyatt, G H, Juniper, E F, Walter, S D, Griffith, L E and Goldstein, R (1998). Interpreting treatment effects in randomised trials. *British Medical Journal* **316**:690–3.

Haskell, W L (1994). Health consequences of physical activity: understanding and challenges regarding dose–response. *Medicine and Science in Sports and Exercise* **26**(6):649–60.

Health Education Authority (1996). *Promoting physical activity through primary health care: guidance for the primary healthcare team.* London: Health Education Authority.

Health Education Authority and Sports Council (1992). *Allied Dunbar National Fitness Survey.* London: Health Education Authority.

Hillsdon, M and Thorogood, M (1996). A systematic review of physical activity promotion strategies. *British Journal of Sports Medicine* **30**:84–9.

Hillsdon, M, Thorogood, M, Anstiss, T and Morris, J (1995). Randomised controlled trials of physical activity promotion in free-living populations: a review. *Journal of Epidemiology and Community Health* **49**:448–53.

ICRF Oxcheck study group (1994). Effectiveness of health checks conducted by nurses in primary care: results of the OXCHECK study after one year. *British Medical Journal* **308**:308–12.

ICRF Oxcheck study group (1995): Effectiveness of health checks conducted by nurses in primary care: final results of the OXCHECK study. *British Medical Journal* **310**:1099–104.

Iliffe, S, See Tai, S, Gould, M, Thorogood, M and Hillsdon, M (1994). Prescribing exercise in general practice. *British Medical Journal* **309**:494–5.

King, A C, Blair, S N, Bild, D E, Dishman, R K, Dubbert, P M and Marcus, B H (1992). Determinants of physical activity and interventions in adults. *Medicine and Science in Sports and Exercise* **24**:S221–S226.

King, A C, Jeffery, R W, Fridinger, F, Dusenbury, L, Provence, S, Hedlund, S A and Spangler, K (1995). Environmental and policy approaches to cardiovascular disease prevention through physical activity: issues and opportunities. *Health Education Quarterly* **22**(4):499–511.

Kreuter, M W, Scharff, D C, Brennan, L K and Lukwago, S N (1997). Physician recommendations for diet and physical activity. *Preventive Medicine* **26**:825–33.

Lewis, B S and Lynch, W D (1993). The effect of physician advice on exercise behavior. *Preventive Medicine* **22**:110–21.

Lord, J C and Green, F (1995). Exercise on prescription: does it work? *Health Education Journal* **54**:453–64.

Mant, J, Dawes, M and Graham-Jones, S (1996). Internal validity of trials is more important than generalisability. *British Medical Journal* **312**:779.

Marcus, B H (1995). Exercise behavior and strategies for intervention. *Research Quarterly for Exercise and Sport* **66**(4):319–23.

Marcus, B H, Goldstein, M G, Jette, A, Simkin-Silverman, L, Pinto, B M, Milan, F, Washburn, R, Smith, K, Rakowski, W and Dube, C E (1997). Training physicians to conduct physical activity counseling. *Preventive Medicine* **26**:382–8.

Marcus, B H, Pinto, B M, Clark, M M, DePue, J D, Goldstein, M G and Silverman, L S (1995). Physician-delivered physical activity and nutrition interventions. *Medicine, Exercise Nutrition and Health* **4**:325–34.

Marcus, B H, Rossi, J S, Selby, V C, Niaura, R S and Abrams, D B (1992). The stages and processes of exercise adoption and maintenance in a worksite sample. *Health Psychology* **11**:386–95.

McDowell, N, McKenna, J and Naylor, P-J (1997). Factors that influence practice nurses to promote physical activity. *British Journal of Sports Medicine* **31**:308–13.

Morris, J N (1994). Exercise in the prevention of coronary heart disease: today's best buy in public health. *Medicine and Science in Sport and Exercise* **26**:838–43.

Munro, J (1997). A randomised controlled trial of exercise in over-65-years-olds: experience from the first year. In Huber, Dr G (ed.), *Proceedings of the 4th International Conference on Physical Activity, Ageing and Sports*: 264–7. Hamburg: Health Promotion Publications.

Murphy, M H and Hardman, A E (1998). Training effects of short and long bouts of brisk walking in sedentary women. *Medicine and Science in Sports and Exercise* **30**(1):152–7.

NHS Centre for Reviews and Dissemination (1996). *Undertaking systematic reviews of research on effectiveness*. CRD report 4. York: NHS Centre for Reviews and Dissemination.

Naylor, P J, Simmonds, G, Riddoch, C, Velleman, G and Turton, P (in press). Improving exercise behavior: the effectiveness of stages of change based advice in the primary care setting.

Nichol, J P (1994). Health and healthcare costs and benefits of exercise. *PharmocoEconomics* **5**(2):109–22.

Paffenbarger, R S J, Hyde, R T, Wing, A L, Lee, I M, Jung, D L and Kampert, J B (1993). The association of changes in physical activity level and other lifestyle characteristics with mortality among men. *New England Journal of Medicine* **328**(8):538–45.

Pate, R R, Pratt, M, Blair, S N, Haskell, W L, Macera, C A, Bouchard, C, Buchner, D, Ettinger, W, Heath, G W, King, A C, Kriska, A, Leon, A S, Marcus, B H, Morris, J, Paffenbarger, Jr., Patrick, K, Polock, M L, Rippe, J M, Sallis, J and Wilmore, J H (1995). Physical activity and Public Health. *Journal of the American Medical Association* **273**(5):402–7.

Powell, K E, Kreuter, M W, Stephens, T, Marti, B and Heinemann, L (1991). The dimensions of health promotion applied to physical activity. *Journal of Public Health Policy*, Winter: 492–509.

Powell, K E, Thompson, P D, Caspersen, C J and Kendrick, K S (1987). Physical activity and the incidence of coronary heart disease. *Annual Review of Public Health* **8**:281–7.

Prentice, A M and Jebb, S A (1995). Obesity in Britain: gluttony or sloth? *British Medical Journal* **311**:437–9.

Pringle, M and Churchill, R (1995). Randomised controlled trials in general practice. *British Medical Journal* **311**:1382–3.

Prochaska, J O and DiClemente, C C (1983). Stages and processes of self change in smoking: towards an integrative model of change. *Journal of Consulting and Clinical Psychology* **51**:390–5.

Redman, S (1996). Towards a research strategy to support public health programs for behaviour change. *Australian and New Zealand Journal of Public Health* **20**(4):352–8.

Riddoch, C J, Vernon, D, Hanbury, A, Simonds, G and Naylor, P J (forthcoming). Exercise promotion in primary care: results of a controlled trial.

Rollnick, S, Kinnersley, P and Stott, N (1993). Methods of helping patients with behaviour change. *British Medical Journal* **307**:188–90.

South Thames Regional Health Authority (1994). *The development of effective evaluation for health promotion activity within the new GP contract*. London: South Thames Regional Health Authority.

Speller, V, Learmonth, A and Harrison, D (1997). The search for evidence of effective health promotion. *British Medical Journal* **315**:361–3.

Stevens, W, Hillsdon, M, Thorogood, M and McArdle, D (forthcoming). The cost effectiveness of a primary-care based physical activity intervention in 45–74 year old men and women: a randomised controlled trial. *British Journal of Sports Medicine*.

Swinburn, B A, Walter, L G, Arroll, B, Tilyard, M W and Russell, D G (1998). The Green Prescription Study: a randomized controlled trial of written exercise advice provided by general practitioners. *American Journal of Public Health* **88**(2):288–91.

Taylor, A H (1996). Evaluating GP exercise referral schemes: findings from a randomised control study. Chelsea School Topic Report No. 6, University of Brighton.

Taylor, A H, Doust, J and Webborn, N (1998). Randomised controlled trial to examine the effects of a GP exercise referral programme in Hailsham, East Sussex, on modifiable coronary heart disease factors. *Journal of Epidemiology and Community Health*.

Tudor-Smith, C, Nutbeam, D, Moore, L and Catford, J (1998). Effects of the Heartbeat Wales programme over five years on behavioural risks for cardiovascular disease: quasi-experimental comparison of results from Wales and a matched reference area. *British Medical Journal* **316**:818–22.

Vernon, D (1994). Effectiveness of a GP-referral scheme in modifying the stage of behaviour change, physical activity and self-efficacy for exercise. MSc thesis, University of Bristol, Bristol.

Webborn, A D J (1996). Systematic review of physical activity promotion strategies. *British Journal of Sports Medicine* **30**:268.

Wiesemann, A, Metz, J, Nuessel, E, Scheidt, R and Scheuermann, W (1997). Four years of practice-based and exercise-supported behavioural medicine in one community of the German CINDI area. *International Journal of Sports Medicine* **18**(4):308–15.